T0258543

Brain Tumor: An Integrated Study

Brain Tumor:
An Integrated Study

Edited by **Michael Jones**

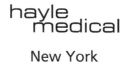

New York

Published by Hayle Medical,
30 West, 37th Street, Suite 612,
New York, NY 10018, USA
www.haylemedical.com

Brain Tumor: An Integrated Study
Edited by Michael Jones

International Standard Book Number: 978-1-63241-064-1 (Hardback)

Printed in the United States of America.

Contents

Permissions

List of Contributors

Preface

This book has been a concerted effort by a group of academicians, researchers and scientists, who have contributed their research works for the realization of the book. This book has materialized in the wake of emerging advancements and innovations in this field. Therefore, the need of the hour was to compile all the required researches and disseminate the knowledge to a broad spectrum of people comprising of students, researchers and specialists of the field.

In the past few years, a remarkable increase in knowledge of microscopic study of brain tumors has been witnessed. Treatments like angiogenesis and immunotherapy have also been tagged important. Along with this, new pathways leading to detailed study and importance of stem cells and microRNAs have been made. Detailed information about the reaction of tumors to chemotherapy and radiation therapy has been provided. Tumors, which are a challenge to humankind, can be combated with new effectual regimen methods. This book provides an insight into up-to-date information related to novel anticancer agents, MicroRNAs, pediatric brain tumors, radio resistance of brain tumors and stem cells.

At the end of the preface, I would like to thank the authors for their brilliant chapters and the publisher for guiding us all-through the making of the book till its final stage. Also, I would like to thank my family for providing the support and encouragement throughout my academic career and research projects.

Editor

Novel Anticancer Agents

A Rational for Novel Anti-NeuroOncology Drugs

Lee Roy Morgan

Additional information is available at the end of the chapter

1. Introduction

Glioblastoma multiforme (GBM) is the most prevalent and lethal type of primary central nervous system tumors with a medium survival of 10-12 months, even with aggressive surgery, radiation and advanced chemotherapy [1]. Poor prognosis of patients with GBM has recently been connected with elevated expressions of a sphingosine kinase [2].

Although, GBM is an extremely lethal cancer, metastatic cancers to the brain from other organs are the most common intracranial tumors, out numbering GBM and other primary brain tumors by at least 10-fold [3]. Lung, breast and melanoma are the 1, 2, 3 most common cancers that metastasize to the brain [4]. The prognosis for these patients is worse than for primary CNS malignancies – 3.7 *vs.*10-12 months for GBM [5].

Intracranial tumors, primary as well as metastatic, are increasing at an alarming rate since many patients with excellent quality of life who appear to have 'beaten the odds' develop metastatic disease to the brain after years of remission from breast and other cancers [3-6]. The development of CNS metastasis results in progressive physical and cognitive impairment and culminates in death within a few months of diagnosis.

In the US alone, the incidence of brain metastasis is expected to exceed 200,000 cases in 2012 – more than 20 times the incidence of primary high grade brain tumors. The median survival time for metastatic cancer to the brain is 2-3 months and with aggressive therapy – maybe 4-12 months [6]!

Over the past 25 years, approximately 4-25 MM cancer patients have died with brain metastasis! These staggering facts strengthen a plea for developing new treatments for both primary and secondary cancers of the brain.

There are many reasons so few drugs are available to treat CNS cancers. Classically patients with brain metastasis have been excluded from clinical trials because of their poor prognosis; the FDA has always had concerns regarding patient safety during Phase I trials with unknown drugs that may cause CNS toxicity and finally once a new drug is identified to have activity in non-CNS cancer involvement, few sponsors want to risk the potential hazards of toxicity that could result from treating patients with CNS involvement – primary or metastatic. Thus, there have been limited attempts to develop drugs for patients with brain metastasis, as well as primary brain tumors. The problem has been compounded by the lack of attention to CNS drug distribution and penetration of brain tumors, with reduction in toxicities.

Thus, there is a major need for the development of unique anticancer molecules that are able to cross the blood brain barrier (BBB), initiate anticancer activity in the CNS tumors and are non-neurotoxicity.

2. Landscape analysis of drugs available for brain tumors

- **Temodar** (temozolamide, TMZ (Schering-Plough,) is currently approved and marketed by Schering-Plough for the treatment of high-grade glioblastoma multiforme and refractory anaplastic astrocytoma in both in combination with radiation.

- **Gliadel** (BCNU wafer, Eisai) is an implantable wafer also used for the treatment of primary brain tumors.

- **Avastin** (bevacizumab, Genentech/Roche) is an anti-angiogenic inhibitor that is being combined with other agents that can penetrate the BBB. Combinations such as *Avastin* plus *Camptosar* (*irinotecan/CPT-11*) +/- *Temodar* are in trials.

- **Tarceva** (erlotinib, OSI Pharmaceuticals), was granted FDA orphan drug designation in August 2003 for patients with malignant gliomas, a recent study of Tarceva found 16% of patients with malignant gliomas who were given Tarciva alone or in combination with Temodar showed tumor shrinkage. The main side effect was an acne-like rash.

- **Iressa** (gefitinib, AstraZeneca) and has been approved for relapsing non-small cell lung cancer. A recent phase II trial of Iressa in patients with relapsed glioblastoma resulted in one of 52 patients achieving a partial response and 22 patients achieving stable disease. Side effects were limited to rash and diarrhea.

- **Zarnestra** (tipifarnib, Johnson & Johnson Pharmaceutical) is in early phase trials for brain tumors. The drug is also being studied in patients with leukemia and breast or lung cancers.

- **81C6** is a tenascin radioactive monoclonal antibody that is injected into a cavity created by the neurosurgeon after removal of the tumor. The antibodies deliver radiation to kill the tumor cells with less radiation to normal brain tissue than conventional radiotherapy. The product is under development at Duke Comprehensive Cancer Center.

- **BMS-247550** (Bristol Myers Squibb) is in Phase II/III @ Memorial Sloan-Kettering.

- **Ipilimumab** (yervoy, Bristol Myers Squibb) a monoclonal antibody to CTLA-4 has activity in melanoma with improved PFS.

- **Vemurafenib** (zelboraf, Genentech) is a BRAF inhibitor approved to treat melanoma, however, CNS mets were excluded in the trials, so the drug is being checked formally now.

- Cisplatin + etoposide, capecitabine (Xeloda), etc. – TTP/PFS - 3 mos max

- Dabrafenib and trametinib have delayed melanoma progression (GlaxoSmithKline)

- And others .... [7-9]

3. A new approach to new novel agents for – 1° and 2° brain tumors

The current trend to develop 'personalized therapy' based on the presence of specific phenotypic or genotypic pathways is an improved approach over the structure activity relationships (SAR) of the 20th century medicinal chemists [10]. However, the management of unresectable brain tumors has not improved. There is still a deficit in drugs that cross the blood brain barrier (BBB), are not recycled out of the brain, are effective anticancer agents in the CNS and do not require hepatic activation. Most of the 21st century 'personalized medicine' drugs are large molecules that are given with other drugs and are ionizable chemicals that cannot penetrate the BBB and/or recycled out of the brain.

A suggested platform for new novel agents – that might be effective therapies for brain tumors comes from the earlier 20th century literature that focused on – '*the energy of cancer cells vs. normal cells*' [11-13].

Brain tumor biochemistry began in 1930 with Warburg's publication - *The Metabolism of Tumors* [12]. The fundamental finding of this publication was that embryonic and tumor tissues have in common a high glycolytic metabolism even under aerobic conditions; in contrast to most normal tissue where oxidative metabolism predominates. The oxidative metabolism in cells is generally 16 x more economical in respect to energy than the glycolytic pathway. The Embden-Meyerhof glycolytic pathway is phylogenetically the more primitive form [12]. *In rapidly growing de-differentiated tissue, this pathway prevails over oxidative metabolism.*

These concepts are of interest because the energy for a healthy cell is generated from glucose where 36 ATP molecules are produced from 1 glucose molecule. Hydrolysis of ATP results in a free energy change of ~ -16,000 cal/ATP molecule, depending on the conditions.

Classically cancer cells generate 2 ATP/1 glucose molecule *vs.* 36 ATP/1 glucose molecule (for healthy normal cells) – with the end product of pyruvate, rather than CO_2 and water as occurs in healthy cells [12]. Otto Warburg explained the latter as a result of the cancer cell's energy-transfer conversion to aerobic glycolysis, a major shift in energy available for cellular work [12].

Albert Szent-Gyorgyi referred to the energy differences of cancer cells *vs.* normal cells as – the *alpha* (α) state with ↑ΔS and ↓ΔF *vs.* the *beta* state (β), with ↓ΔS and ↑ΔF), resp. [13].

The α state is the ground state of life! The most stable state of any system is with minimum ΔF and maximum ΔS. If the cellular organization becomes unstable, cells will return to an α state and remain there. The more complete the return – the harder it will be to reverse.

The β state is where there is a high degree of differentiation and potential for release of F if the cells react and initiate differentiation. Here the energy present allow cellular regulation and multicellular organisms replication; not a mass of undifferentiated cells – cancer.

[Where, S = entropy or potential (stored capacity) for a reaction to occur and F (free energy), a state of function depending only on the initial and final states of a system [14].

The importance of ΔF is that the value immediately provides quantitative information about the potential ability of a substance to undergo a chemical or physical transformation. A reaction may proceed spontaneously without external energy only if the ΔF is negative (energy dissipated) [14]. Chemical thermodynamics tells us that *"F needs to be a released in order for the cell to be productive and do work, not just replicate with a low productive reactivity"* [13].

We should view entropy as an index of a condition or character. It is an index of the capacity for spontaneous changes. By historical accident, the index was actually defined so that it *increased* as the capacity of an isolated system for spontaneous change *decreased*.

Hence, entropy is an index of exhaustion. The more a system has lost its capacity for spontaneous change, the greater is the entropy [14].

Yes, cancer cells represent a primitive, high random energy, low functional state with unbridled proliferation [13]. Cancer cells are not sick or weak, their vitality, as a wild type, may be even higher than that of a normal cell.

The cancer cell is unable to rebuild its beta state after it has completed its division and has to persist in the proliferative alpha state until death. In itself, the proliferative state would not be pathological – it is only its timing and irreversibility, which makes it so. *It is not pathological to be an infant, but it is pathological to be one and remain so x 50 years!*

Is cancer an outward manifestation resulting from depletion in cellular free energy within cells and increased entropy?

Although oxygen is considered essential for life, sulfur (S) and phosphorus (P) are the most common biological selections for energy transfer. The latter two elements are members of the Third Period of the Periodic Table and are capable of accepting an additional pair of electrons into unoccupied $3d$ orbitals. This phenomenon is characteristic of the elements of the Third Period, which possess d, in addition to s and p orbitals, and thus have a place to hold electrons beyond the normal outer-shell octet. Molecules that possess P or S can store electrons (energy) and then release the energy during the transfer of shared electrons to other electron deficient molecules [15].

ATP (Fig. 1) is a unique example of how a 3rd Period element - 'P' participates in a key natural energy-rich compound, which upon hydrolysis generates ~ 8 kcal/mole upon hydrolysis with a +ΔF. When hydrolyzed in the presence of suitable transformers (transducing systems), the energy liberated may be used for cellular or tissue processes – cellular metabolism, nerve conduction, cell membrane transport, etc.

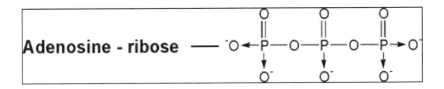

Figure 1. Adenosine triphosphate (ATP)

Energy rich phosphates usually possess either a second phosphoryl group or a resonating organic radical capable of entering into conjugation with the mobile electrons. This type of molecule usually contains a chain of at least three adjacent atoms, all bearing a net positive charge (deficient in π electrons), the chain sometimes extends over a five or even six atoms [Fig. 2], [16].

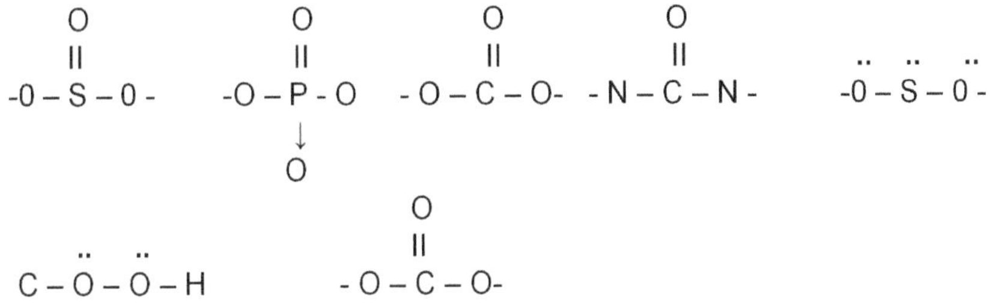

$$
\begin{array}{ccccc}
O & O & O & O & \\
\| & \| & \| & \| & \\
-0-S-0- & -O-P-O & -O-C-O- & -N-C-N- & -0-S-0- \\
& \downarrow & & & \\
& O & & & \\
\end{array}
$$

$$
\begin{array}{cc}
& O \\
& \| \\
C-O-O-H & -O-C-O-
\end{array}
$$

Figure 2. Examples of 3-atom high-energy moieties

Many of the small molecules used as anti-CNS cancer agents also possess 3-atom high energy moieties (in red) [3]

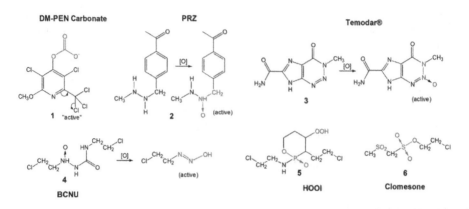

Figure 3. Small Molecules that are used to treat CNS cancer

Where: **DM-PEN carbonate**, 1 is a carbonate analog of 4-demethyl penclomedine; **PRZ**, 2 is dacarbazine; **Temodar®**, 3 is temozolamide (TMZ); **BCNU**, 4 is bis-(chloroethyl)nitrosourea; **HOOI**, 5 is 4-hydroperoxyifosfamide; **Clomesone**, 6 is a chloroethylating agent similar to BCNU – alkylates guanine-O[6] [17].

Compounds can be classified as "energy-rich" or "energy-poor" based on their ΔF. Energy poor compounds do not possess more than two adjacent atoms bearing a positive charge and poorly absorbed by the CNS.

Thus, the design of "high-energy molecules" that are lipophilic, energetic and absorbed into a low free energy (ΔF) and high entropy (ΔS) cancer environment are timely. The latter is a unique therapeutic target – *the result of inefficient energy of cancer cells* [14].

Life is controlled by the transfer of energy. All living systems obey the 1st law of thermo-dynamics – which states that the sum of all energies in an isolated system remains constant. Energy may be converted into another form but the quantity can be neither created nor destroyed [18].

A question to be answered – are high energy compounds really attracted to low energy highly utilized regions in the body?

4. Polyhalogenated pyridyl carbonates [16, 19-21]

The polyhalogenated pyridyl carbonates are neutral molecules that when coupled with lip-ids via high energy linkers – carbonates, phosphates, etc., fulfill the above requirements for novel high energy anticancer agents that could be attracted to and accumulate in CNS can-cer tissue [16, 19-21]. The carbonate moiety like phosphate has the properties (resonance) of the high energy 3-atom moieties described in Fig. 3.

DEKK-TEC has designed a series of polychlorinated pyridyl carbonates (with 1 as a template, Fig. 3) that are linked with lipids and lipophilic moieties to promote CNS penetration [19]. DM-CHOC-PEN (4-demethyl-4-cholesteryloxycarbonylpenclomedine) is the most active and stable member of a large series of carbonates with improved activity vs. intracranially (IC) implanted human xenograft models – U251 and D54 glioblastoma and MX-1 breast cancer [Table 1] [19].

DM-CHOC-PEN is a unique molecule with several functional moieties that enable it to inhibit cancer replication. The structure contains the following moieties of interest:

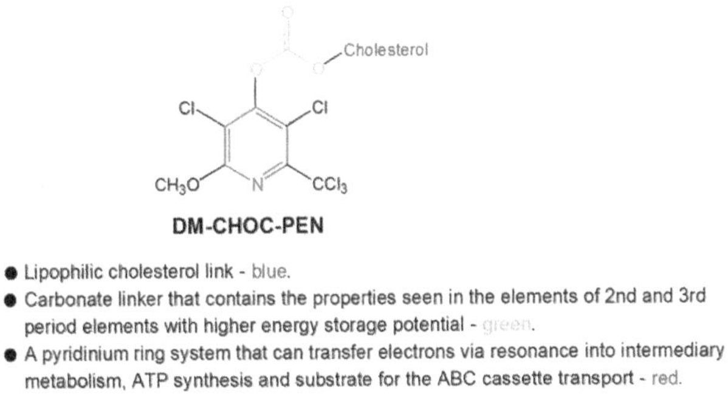

DM-CHOC-PEN

- Lipophilic cholesterol link - blue.
- Carbonate linker that contains the properties seen in the elements of 2nd and 3rd period elements with higher energy storage potential - green.
- A pyridinium ring system that can transfer electrons via resonance into intermediary metabolism, ATP synthesis and substrate for the ABC cassette transport - red.

Figure 4. Lipophilic cholesterol link - blue. Carbonate linker that contains the properties seen in the elements of 2nd and 3rd period elements with higher energz storage potential - green. A pyridinium ring system that can transfer electrons via resonance into intermediary metabolism, ATP synthesis and substrate for the ABC cassette transport / red

The importance of the carbonate moiety is its internal energy and ability to transfer electrons through multiple structures (resonance) (see Fig. 5):

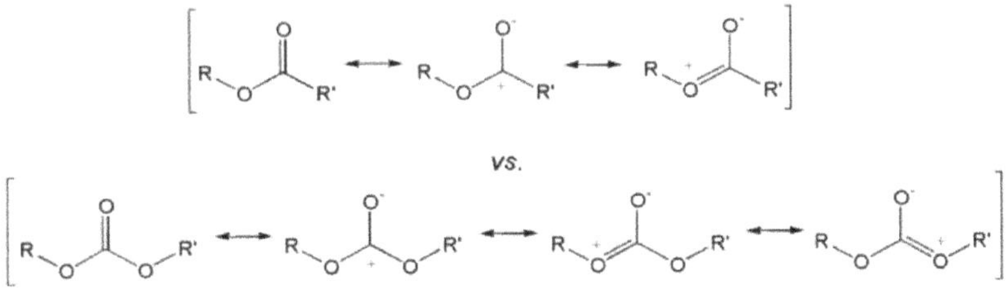

Figure 5. Mesomeric forms of the carbonate; where R = pyridyl group & R'=cholesterol

The additional oxygen in the carbonates [Fig. 5, lower structures] stabilizes the moiety and allows for distribution of charge through resonance (Fig. 5). This chemical property exists in the phosphates and other oxides of the 3rd period elements [see below] [15].

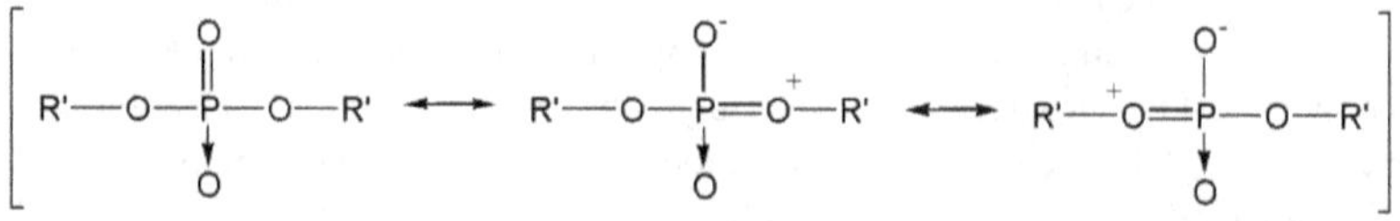

$$\left[\text{R'}-\text{O}-\overset{\overset{\displaystyle \text{O}}{\|}}{\underset{\downarrow}{\text{P}}}-\text{O}-\text{R'} \longleftrightarrow \text{R'}-\text{O}-\overset{\overset{\displaystyle \text{O}^-}{|}}{\underset{\downarrow}{\text{P}}}{=}\overset{+}{\text{O}}-\text{R'} \longleftrightarrow \text{R'}-\overset{+}{\text{O}}{=}\overset{\overset{\displaystyle \text{O}^-}{|}}{\underset{\downarrow}{\text{P}}}-\text{O}-\text{R'} \right]$$

Scheme 1.

In contrast, esters lack the degree of resonance/electron distribution [Fig. 5, upper structures].

As indicated in Fig. 5, a carbonate is not isosteric with an acyl or ester group nor is it a direct extension of an ester group. The carbonate group is unique and when combined with cholesterol its CNS penetration properties are enhanced [Table 1] [16].

	DM-CHOC-PEN			BCNU			TMZ		
Tumor	*Dose	%ILS	%LTS	+Dose	%ILS	%LTS	#Dos	%ILS	%LTS
U251 Glioblastoma	135	+54	+20(1/5 CR)	9	52	+20(1/5 CR)	120	+54	+20(1/5 CR)
D54 Glioblastoma	200	+3	+20(1/5 CR)	NA	NA	NA	NA	NA	NA
MX-1 Breast Cancer	50 100	+20 Toxic	17(1/6 CR)	60	12	0/5	NA	NA	NA

Table 1. Activity of DM-CHOC-PEN vs. Intracerebrally Implanted Xenograft Tumors in Mice

Implant: 10^6 cells IC; Treatment Route: Intraperitoneal (- 5 days post IC implant); Schedule: *IV q1d x 5d; +IV q1d x 3d; #po 1d x 5d; Species: Athymic NCr/nu mice – female, Charles River; Dose: mg/kg; %ILS = % increased life span; %LTS = long term survival; all studies were terminated at 54 days

Based on the preclinical antitumor activities in Table 1, DM-CHOC-PEN produced a moderate increase in life span (% ILS); however it was comparable to that seen with BCNU and TMZ. DM-CHOC-PEN did yield long-term survivors that were healthy with no weight loss. Even the highly resistant IC implanted D54 glioma was sensitive to DM-CHOC-PEN. The drug has minimal toxicity and has encouraging potential [16, 19, 21].

An *in vivo* activation mechanism scheme is shown in Fig. 6, where DM-CHOC-PEN is proposed to be acting as a non-classical alkylating agent. The scheme describes a dual carbonium ion - DNA cross-linking mechanism (in a G-X-C sequence) with tumor DNA in the major groove via N^7- guanine [20]. A bi-molecular coupled product (*via* the trichloromethylene group) has been identified as the major microsomal metabolite of PEN

[20]. The trichloromethylene group is required, since the dichloromethylene analog of PEN is not active [does not react with 4-(p-nitrobenzyl) pyridine (NBP] (Struck, personnel communication).

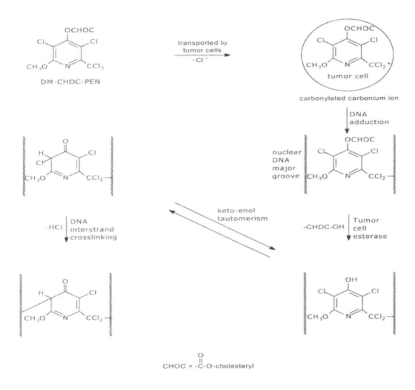

$$CHOC = -\overset{O}{\underset{\|}{C}}-O\text{-cholesteryl}$$

Figure 6. Proposed mechanism of action of 4 - demethyl - 4 - cholesterolyl - penclomedine (DM - CHOC - PEN)

Mice with IC growing U251 gliomas were treated with DM-CHOC-PEN, 135 mg/kg daily x 5-days and after 3-days the animals were sacrificed and the brains with tumors removed. The tumors were easily separated from the normal brain tissue. Each was homogenized in phosphate buffer, extracted with dichloromethane, and evaporated to dryness. The residues were assayed by HPLC and DM-CHOC-PEN, a guanine-N^7-CCl_2-adduct with DM-CHOC-PEN involving the –CCl_3 moiety and the DM-CHCO-PEN dimer-Cl_2C-CCl_2- were identified in the glioma tissue [16]. Neither DM-CHOC-PEN nor metabolites could be identified in the normal brain tissue.

Thus, DM-CHOC-PEN alkylates DNA with adducts at guanine-N^7 that could be quantitated in tumor tissue. The above MOA is in contrast to TMZ, BCNU and others, which alkylate guanine-O^6 [22].

The polyhalogenated pyridyl carbonates are unique structures that cross the BBB, accumulate in CNS tumor tissue, not normal brain tissue and are not recycled out of the CNS are cytotoxic *vs.* intracranially (IC) implanted human tumor xenografts in mouse models; fulfilling all of the criteria of the preceding paragraphs [23].

The combinations of responses in mouse xenograft tumor models, and a lack of neurotoxicity in rat and dog biopsychology studies, have allowed a Phase I trial to be conducted with DM- CHOC-PEN in patients with advanced cancer, including CNS involvement - IND 68,876 [24].

DEKK-TEC and its clinical investigators have satisfied the FDA that they are capable of treating patients with Phase I drugs and diagnosing physical and mental/cognitive alterations that may be associated with CNS tumor growth vs. toxicity secondary to drugs.

5. Phase I clinical trial with a high energy drug – DM-CHOC-PEN

Weiner, Ware, Friedlander, et al. reported preliminary data from a Phase I trial involving 18-patients treated with DM-CHOC-PEN in single IV doses of 39-87.5 mg/m² once every 21-days [25]. Six [6] patients had either CNS or spinal nervous system (SNS) involvement. Most patients had multiple treatments. The longest survivor (a sarcoma w/ SNS involvement) is 19+ months with NED [who also received doxorubicin at a later time] [25].

Support for DM-CHOC-PEN crossing the blood brain barrier in humans is provided from the above trial with reported observations for – GBM, CNS melanoma and breast cancer (BC) having PFS 4-13 mos., objective reductions in tumor sizes and no CNS toxicity.

One patient with pelvic sarcoma spread to the spinal cord required debulking surgery 21-days post treatment with DM-CHOC-PEN (39 mg/m²). Tumor tissue was removed, assayed and DM-CHOC-PEN was quantitated in the spinal sarcoma tissue – 92 ng/g of tumor [25].

The only SLTs noted to date are hyperbilirubinemia in 2-patients with liver metastasis; patients with no liver pathology have not demonstrated SLTs. CNS toxicity has not been noted in any of the patients. Overall, the drug was reported as being tolerated very well [25].

6. CNS melanoma

Melanoma is the third most frequent cancer to metastasize to the brain. It is anticipated that there will be ~ 20,000 new cases of CNS stage melanoma diagnosed in 2012 [9]. Enrollment of these patients with CNS melanoma would be critical to appreciating the activity of the demethylpenclomedine carbonates in this stage of disease [9, 26]. Two of the patients enrolled and treated in the DM-CHOC-PEN Phase I trial had CNS melanoma; one patient had significant shrinkage of CNS lesions, the other stable (NC) disease [25].

To test the potential sensitivity of DM-CHOC-PEN as therapy for melanoma, the B-16 mouse melanoma was selected as a screening model and treated with DM-CHOC-PEN *in vitro* and *in vivo* [28].

7. Experimental methods

In Vitro – B-16 mouse melanoma cells [obtained from ATCC, Menassas, VA] were assayed in culture wells (10^4/mL) using a complete RPMI media containing 10% FBS with pen/strep and maintaining cells @ 36° C in a CO_2 incubator. Drugs (in 1 mL volumes; in conc. - 0.1-5 µg/mL) were added to the cells in a growth phase and removed after 8-12 h; cultures were washed with fresh medium. For florescent studies - cells in growth phase were incubated with dichlorofluorescein diacetate (DCFDA, 3 µg/mL RPMI) x 1-hr, washed and DM-CHOC-PEN added (1-5 µg/mL); incubation continued for an additional 5-hour. Cells were washed with fresh complete media and monitored with fluorescent microscopy. For the latter – RPMI without phenol red was used.

In Vivo – B-16 mouse melanoma cells (10^6) were implanted SC into the flank of adult female C57BL mice (age – 7-9 weeks, Harlan Labs.) and treatments with DM-CHOC-PEN, HOOI, and other drugs began were initiated when lesions were palpable - 3-5 days post implant.

Drugs – were dissolved in saline or in a soybean oil/egg yolk lecithin emulsion (2 mg/mL) and administer by IP injection. HOOI was administered as the L-lysine salt [27].

Results – B-16 cells were incubated with DM-CHOC-PEN and after ~ 6-8 hours became heavily melanotic, lost adherence and floated to the top of the wells. Isolation of the floating heavily pigmented melanotic cells that formed (Fig. 7b), followed by washing, extraction with dichloromethane, and HPLC assays revealed that the cells contained DM-CHOC-PEN in concentrations of 0.003-0.09 µg/mL of packed B-16 cells. Attached amelanotic cells contained 0-20 ng/mL of DM-CHOC-PEN (significant) [28].

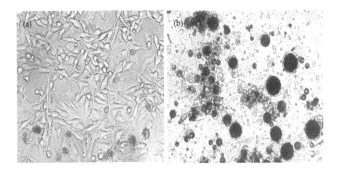

Figure 7. a) B-16 melanoma cells – untreated; b) After treatment with DM-CHOC-PEN

In comparison with other agents – DM-CHOC-PEN had an IC_{50} of 0.4 µg/mL and TMZ, BCNU, DOX and actinomycin D (Act D), HOOI – 0.5-0.9 µg/mL; *cis*-platinum (*cis*-platin) – 1.5 µg/mL resulted in IC_{50} cell death @ 36 hour post-intial exposure. With the exception of DM-CHOC-PEN, all treated cells died with ghosts remaining; excesive melanin formation only occurred with DM-CHOC-PEN; the terminal pathways were quite different for the other drugs.

Drug	IC_{50} (µg/mL)
DM-CHOC-PEN	0.4 +/- 0.01
Actinomycin D	0.5 +/- 0.02
BCNU	0.9 +/- 0.1
cis-Platin	1.5 +/- 0.1
DOX	0.7 +/- 0.1
TMZ	"/>3.0
HOOI	0.8 +/- 0.2

Table 2. Drugs Responses vs. B-16 Melanoma (IC_{50})

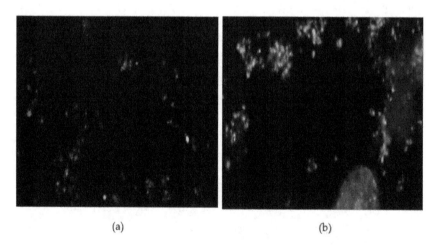

(a)   (b)

Figure 8. a)B-16 cells + DCF-DA; b)B-26 cells plus DM-CHOC-PEN + DCF-DA

Viewed with florescent microscopy – green florescent cells are generating ROS and the DCF is florescent.

Melanoma cell death due to DM-CHOC-PEN could be a result of increased intracellular melanin, as well as DNA alkylation. Addition of DCF-DA (dichlorofluorescein diacetate) to the culture medium (10 µg/mL) documented the formation of radical oxygen species (ROS) in the DM- CHOC-PEN treated cultures; green labeled cells (Fig. 8b). ROS release was documented with DCF, which is due to the hydrolysis and oxidized of DCF-DA by ROS with the release of fluorescent DCF. The generation of ROS was not observed with B-16 melanoma cells treated with *cis*-platin or actinomycin D and cultured under similar conditions. There is some back ground florescence and secondary to melanin-associated ROS formation [16].

In Vivo Studies – Adult female C57BL mice in groups of 5-6 mice with palpable SC nodules were dosed IP daily (175 or 200 mg/kg) for 5-days with DM-CHOC-PEN and monitored daily until death (Fig. 9a).

Mice treated with DM-CHOC-PEN (200 mg/kg/d x 5 days, IP) alone demonstrated an ILS of 142% (Fig. 9a). No drug related toxicity was noted – weight gain occurred until tumor growth was obvious.

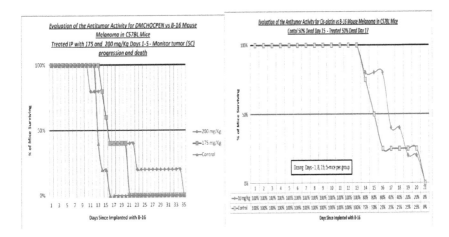

Figure 9. a)DM-CHOC-PEN treated; b)Cis-platin treated

Cis-platin was used as a drug control and administered (IP) once weekly x 3 (Fig. 9b); animals did not tolerate 3- or 5-day dosing schedules [28, 29]. Although active *in vitro, cis*-platin does not improve *in vivo* survival – as seen in Fig. 9b, although it is used in many melanoma clinical protocols [3].

Tumor histology of the DM-CHOC-PEN treated B-16 melanomas are reviewed in Fig. 10. On the left (a) is the saline control and right (b) the DM-CHOC-PEN treated – 200 mg/kg IP daily x 5 days. *Note* - the melanin deposits in the cells with vacuoles, similar to what was seen in culture [29].

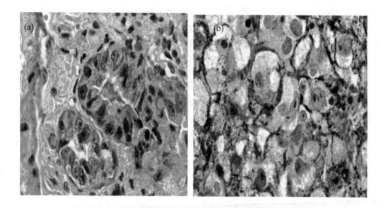

Figure 11. a)Histology of saline controls; b)Histology of DM-CHOC-PEN treated

Tumor tissue from the above DM-CHOC-PEN treated mice were assayed per cytoflorimetry using a BD FAC Scanner.

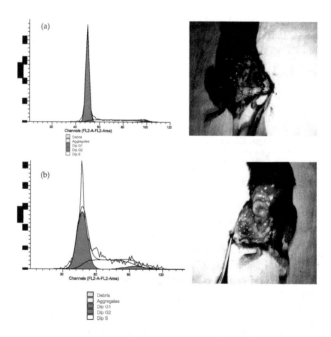

Figure 12. a) Mice bearing SC nodules – control animals. b) Mice bearing SC nodules dosed - 200 mg/kg; days 1-5 and sacrificed 3-days after the last treatment.

There were less viable cells available in the treated animals. DM-CHOC-PEN reduced the cellular concentration of the tumors and the cells accumulated in G_1 phase, with an inhibition in S-phase concentration of cells (Fig. 11b). Thus, more support for DM-CHOCPEN's potential use in melanoma. Unfortunately, there was a significant amount of debris present.

Discussion – Mice bearing B-16 melanoma, tolerated DM-CHOC-PEN well when administered IP daily x 5 days or days 1 & 5 with improved overall survival (OAS) for both schedules; the former was the superior.

Histological examinations of the melanoma tissue from animals that had been treated with DM-CHOC-PEN revealed tumor cells encompassed in extracellular melanin, very similar to what was seen in tissue culture (Fig. 7b). DM-CHOC-PEN was extracted in up to 92 ng/g tissue quantities from the melanoma tissue removed in Fig. 11b [16].

DM-CHOC-PEN is a pseudo-alkylator that binds to DNA's guanine-N^7 via the trichloromethyl moiety → dichloromethylene carbonium ion and can form DNA-guanine adducts and cell death [Fig. 6] [9]. However, the current observations in a melanoma model support DM-CHOC-PEN's additional ability to disrupt cellular metabolism with death via autooxidation of DOPA to melanin and superoxide formation – an additional MOA for consideration – Fig. 12 [28, 29].

Electronic modeling studies support DM-CHOC-PEN's ability to act as a pyridinium co-factor oxidized by the pyridine nucleotides (NAD, etc.) with red-ox transfer of electrons from 3,4-dihydroxyphenylalanine (DOPA) to the mitochondria and cytochrome C/cytochrome oxidase transport system (Fig. 13). This result is the formation of 5, 6-indolequinone and melanin with a trail of electrons that can enter the mitochondrion intermediary pool resulting in all the same type of lethal changes seen with electron beam therapy for cancer [30, 31].

The 'melanin balls' that were seen *in vitro* are spheres of extracellular melanin polymer encapsulating colonies of melanoma cells that could induce a hostile microenvironment through ROS formation with death via oxidative stress and apoptosis (Figs. 10) [30]. Clusters of melanin laden cells contained significantly elevated concentrations of DM-CHOC-PEN, as compared to the amelanotic variant; a possible storage site for the drug [31]. The initial DOPA → DOPA quinone transformation is catalyzed by tyrosinase (DOPA oxidase) intracellular [32-35]. However, the red-ox potential for DM-CHOC-PEN is sufficient to catalyze the conversion with excess melanin formation per the Rapier Scheme below [32].

Both malignant and benign melanocytes generate melanin pigment via the sequence of chemical reactions as depicted in the classical Rapier Scheme in Fig.12 [32].

Melanin is far from being an end-product of oxidation [34-37]. At a glance the existence of energy bands are obvious from the highly conjugated heterocyclic indole quinone structure for melanin (Fig. 12). The hypothesis has been proposed that non-localized empty molecular orbitals are associated with the copolymer chain of the indole quinoid units and that the melanin polymer acts as a one-dimensional semi-conductor/trap with bound protons producing electron traps in the system [36].

Thus, melanin is a polymer of indole-5, 6-quinone which is highly electrophilic due to its conjugated structure and capable of attracting, storing and/or transferring electrons as electrical energy [30, 31, 34]. DM-CHOC-PEN treatment induced ROS formation *via* the melanin system resulting in cancer cell death – an end point.

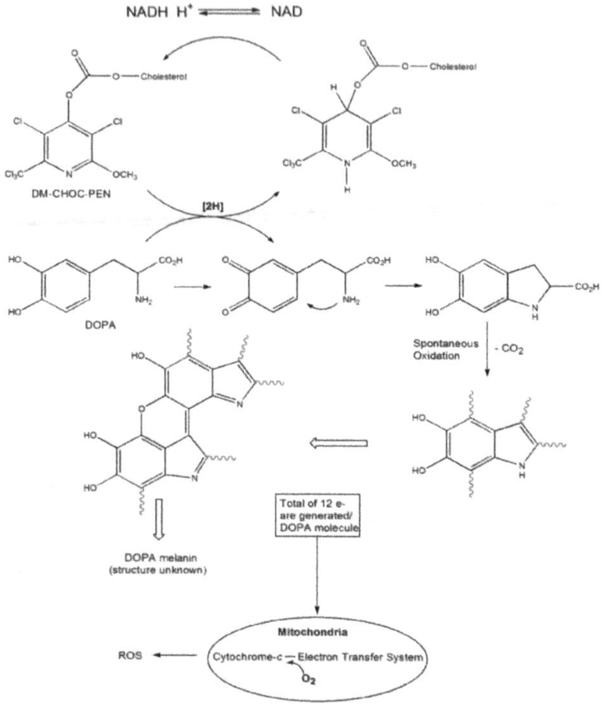

Figure 13. Interaction of DM-CHOC-PEN with Rapier melanin cell cycle and mitochondrion [32]

Melanin is potentially a storage deposit of electrons and/or for electron-rich molecules (reported by our group years ago) [31]. Due to the high redox potential between DOPA and DOPA quinone, +0.37v, a possible yield of -19.8 kcal/mole occurs upon the oxidation of 1 mole DOPA. A total of 12 e$^-$ are generated per mole of DOPA oxidized to indole quinone which polymerize to melanin [Fig. 13 [31]. A field of melanin encompassing a colony of cancer cells could generate a hostile electrical microenvironment and inhibit cellular metabolism and replication [33].

Melanoma cells are a classical representation of cancer cells with a resting low free energy (ΔF) and high entropy (ΔS) – the *alpha state* [14]. The interactions of DM-CHOC-PEN and DOPA induced the formation of melanin and ROS which resulted in an increased environmental ΔF and a decrease in ΔS; a new resting high energy state – the *beta state*. The cells that are contained in the melanin balls are in a *beta state* - undergo apoptosis and die [28, 30, 31].

Thus, DM-CHOC-PEN is a new drug entity that crosses the BBB and couples two new targets – the melanin cycle and superoxide formation with apoptosis plus DNA guanine – N^7 adducts. DM-CHOC-PEN is a potential triple treat for CNS melanoma, the 3rd most common cancer that spreads to the CNS.

8. A 2nd High energy drug

Another high energy drug, 4-hydroperoxyifosfamide (HOOI) [Fig. 3, 14] and is a pre-activated form of ifosfamide (IFOS) which possesses the criteria for discussion [Fig. 14]. HOOI also contains a 3rd Period atom – 'P'; thus it has two centers of high energy – Fig 3, 14.

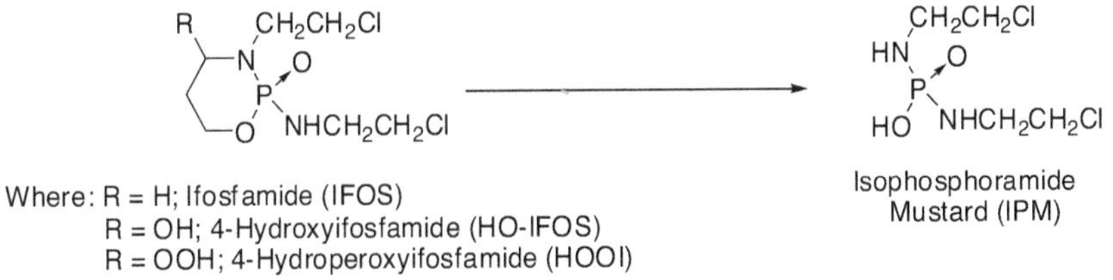

Where: R = H; Ifosfamide (IFOS)
    R = OH; 4-Hydroxyifosfamide (HO-IFOS)
    R = OOH; 4-Hydroperoxyifosfamide (HOOI)

Isophosphoramide
Mustard (IPM)

Figure 14. Ifosfamide and analogs

IFOS is a well-known anticancer agent that requires hepatic activation to 4-HO-IFOS which spontaneously undergoes hydrolysis with ring opening resulting in isophosphoramide mustard (IPM) [Fig. 14], the latter is the active cytotoxic form of IFOS [37-39]. As part of the IFOS activation process, hepatic metabolic dechloroethylation releases chloroacetaldehyde, which has been proposed to be the major cause of IFOS associated neurotoxicity [40]. Acrolein is also released and has been implicated in dose limiting toxicities - hemorrhagic cystitis and 2° tumor promotion [41-45].

In contrast, HOOI does not require hepatic microsomal activation, crosses the BBB and is readily absorbed by cancer cells where it releases IPM *in situ* [46, 47]. The former does not generate chloroacetaldehyde (neurotoxic) during its conversion to IPM, as does IFOS. Neither hemorrhagic cystitis nor renal toxicity has been observed with HOOI in animal toxicology models. Pulmonary damage that could occur with peroxides – pulmonary air emboli was not observed in the dog HOOI study [46]. Hematological toxicity (bone marrow depletion) was the dose limiting toxicity in the dog study [47].

The potential therapeutic usefulness of HOOI is supported by in vivo activity in human tumor xenografts and cyclophosphamide (CPA)-resistant murine tumor models plus reduced toxicities.

In vivo in comparison to CPA and IFOS in rodent and dog species [Table 3] [47], a potentially improved safety profile is anticipated – with reduced systemic formation of acrolein and the absence of chloroacetaldehyde during the conversion of HOOI to IPM – *in situ* [47].

Drug	Dose (mg/kg/day)	No of Mice	MX-1* T- C (Days)	ZR-75-1* T- C (Days)	U251 (%ILS)**	P388/CPA (% ILS)**
HOOI	90 (<LD$_{10}$)	10	>28.8 9 (33% LTS)	>46.1 (83% CR)	+54 (1/5 CR)	+209+
DM-CHOC-PEN	135	10	>54 days (20% LTS) [Dose - 50]	NA	+54 (1/5 CR)	NA
IFOS	40 (MTD)++	10	8.6 (7% LTS)	>43.8 (17% CR)	50 (0/5 CR)	42
IPM	40 (MTD)++	10	2.1	NA	NA	+85
BCNU	9-15 (MTD)	5	12% LTS; 0 CR	NA	+52 (1/5 CR)	NA
TMZ	120 mg (MTD)	5	NA	NA	+54 (1/5 CR)	NA

Dose – qd x 5d (IP) – except TMZ – PO Q4D x 3; *human breast cancer – SC implanted, **human glioblastoma – IC implanted; ***CPA (cyclophosphamide) – resistant murine leukemia. For MX-1 – T-C (days) = difference in median times post implant for tumors of treated groups to attain an evaluation size compared to median of control group; +6-log cell kill; ++>40 mg/kg was too toxic; ***% ILS (increased length of survival – study terminated @ 54 days.

Table 3. Human Xenografts and Murine Tumors Growing in Mouse Models

HOOI possesses two [2] 3-high energy atom chains, thus the drug more than fits the criteria proposed earlier in this chapter (3). In addition, HOOI does not require activation by the liver and spontaneously undergoes conversion to IPM and cross-links with nuclear DNA via major groove alkylation – N^7-guanine, forming G-X-C adducts [39].

Of significance is that HOOI was curative (54% LTS, with 20% CR) *vs.* the human U251 glioblastoma implanted IC as well as the MX-1 breast cancer IC model (Table 3) [47]. It should also be noted that BCNU – the gold standard for years in the treatment of gliomas produced no CRs and TMZ the current standard produced identical responses to HOOI.

Like DM-CHOC-PEN, HOOI accumulates in U-251 glioma tissue in 50 ng/g tissue content when the drug is administered IP to animals bearing IC implanted tumors [47]. No CNS/behavioral alterations or toxicity have been noted for HOOI [48].

Unlike ifosfamide (IFOS), HOOI is more lipophilic, activated *in situ*, with less extracellular acrolein, no chloroacetaldehyde released and no IFOS associated CNS or GU toxicity [48]. In dogs the principal toxicity with HOOI was bone marrow suppression that reversed with time [47, 48].

An early study reported that SK-MEL-31 human melanoma cells were sensitive to HOOI, which prompted the comparison of the drug with DM-CHOC-PEN in the B-16 melanoma model [47].

In 2012, the incidence of new cases of melanoma in the US alone is estimated at 76,250, an increase of ~ 20% during the past 10 years [9]. Of these cases, ~ 25% will metastasize to the CNS; thus our interest in the drug [26].

Fig. 15 describes the impact on survival of B-16 mouse melanoma when HOOI is administered alone and with DM-CHOC-PEN [49].

DM-CHOC-PEN (200 mg/kg/d) was injected IP daily x 5-days followed by HOOI (90 mg/m²) IP daily x 3 days (Day 6-8). The latter is a more classical mustard type agent with activity in the G_1 phase, as compared to DM-CHOC-PEN, which inhibited cell replication at the S phase – Fig. 12b [49].

The %LTS for the 2-drug combination was 173% vs. HOOI alone - 78%; for DM-CHOC-PEN alone - 142% (see Fig. 14).

No drug related toxicity was noted – weight gain continued until tumor growth was a burden and animals sacrificed. The use of 5-day dosing for HOOI was toxic and not considered [48].

Combination of the two -'high energy' agents selected for discussion as binary therapy has potential. It will be a while before these 2-drugs are administered together; however, other binary selections that incorporate DM-CHOC-PEN are in the planning stage for Phase II trials.

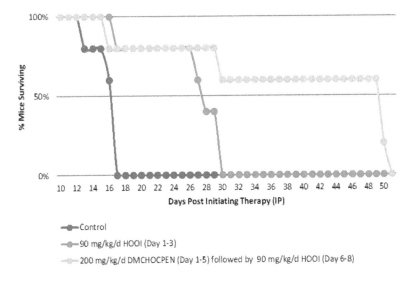

Figure 15. DM-CHOC-PEN plus HOOI in the Treatment of B-16 Mouse Melanoma

9. Conclusion

Melanoma cells, as seen in Fig. 7a represent classical cancer cells with a resting low free energy (ΔF) and high entropy (ΔS) – the *alpha state* [14]. The interaction of DM-CHOC-PEN and DOPA induced the formation of melanin – a high energy component/storage that resulted in an increase in environmental ΔF and a decrease in ΔS; a new resting high energy state – the *beta state* [14]. Cells that are encompassed in the 'melanin balls' (Fig. 7b) were converted to a well differentiated state and die. The addition of HOOI to DM-CHOC-PEN inhibited those cells that reversed to the *alpha state* – survive and continue to replicate. Thus, the binary combination improved %LTS vs. either drug alone; supporting the *in vitro* observations.

Although, only two patients with CNS melanoma have been treated with DM-CHOC-PEN in the Phase I trial, the report that one patient did demonstrate an interval response and one patent had a no change response, both with no neurotoxicity is encouragement for the potential use of the drug in the treatment of CNS melanoma [25]. HOOI has not been used in clinical trials as yet.

There are many novel drugs that fall in to the 'high-energy' category that should be evaluated or re-visited. In particular – clomesone [Fig. 3], a drug developed at Southern Research Institute, US had potential in animal studies, but produced hematological toxicity in Phase I trials and discontinued from studies [17, 50]. The drug has novel chloroethylating properties and like BCNU forms adducts with DNA guanine-O^6 [50]. In addition, the drug contains two - S - atoms which are a 3rd Period element and able to expand its 3d orbital – a real 'high-energy' molecule. However, only one of the latter groups has the ability to resonant with energy storage.

With the two sets of 3-atom chain as a point of interest (Fig. 3, 6), clomesone should be revisited with dose modifications; it has potential [52].

In summary, three 'high energy' drugs have been reviewed as support that a novel approach to the treatment of CNS malignancies could be through the inefficient energy system of brain tumors [11, 12]. Anticancer agents that have the appropriate structure, can penetrate the CNS, not be recycled out and inhibit cancer growth.

Over all, DM-CHOC-PEN has been well tolerated in Phase I studies with advanced –breast cancer, sarcoma, glioblastoma multiforme, melanoma, pancreas, esophageal, non-small cell lung cancer colorectal cancer and cervical cancer and will obviously enter Phase II trials alone or as binary therapy [25].

Furthermore, HOOI is being readied for Phase I clinical trials and the results should be equally interesting.

Acknowledgement

Grant support from NCI/SBIR R43/44CA85021 and R43CA132257 is appreciated.

The author wishes to thank Drs. Robert F. Struck, Branko S. Jursic, Roy S. Weiner, Marcus L. Ware, Barry Sartin, Philip Friedlander, Andrew Rodgers and Mr. Edmund Benes for their discussions, review and comments during the preparation of this manuscript.

Author details

Lee Roy Morgan*

Address all correspondence to: LRM1579@aol.com

CEO DEKK-TEC, Inc University of New Orleans New Orleans, LA, USA

References

[1] Maher, EA, Furnari, FB, Bachoo, RM, et al. Malignant glioblastoma: genetics and biology of a grave matter. Genes Dev., 15:1311-33, 2001.

[2] Van Brachlyn, JR, Jackson, CA, Pearl, DK, et al. Spingosine kinase -1 expression correlates with poor survival of patients with GBM: roles of spingosine kinase isoforms in glioblastoma cell lines. J. Neuropatol. Exp. Neurol, 64: 695-705, 2005.

[3] Patchell, RA. The management of brain metastasis. Cancer Treatment Rev. 29: 533-40.

[4] Johnson, JD, Young, B, Demographics of brain metastasis. Neurosurg. Clin. N. Am., 7: 337-44, 1996.

[5] Sampson, JH, Carter, JH, Friedman, AH, Seiger, HF. Demographics, prognosis and therapy in 702 patients with brain metastasis from malignant melanoma. J. Neurosurg., 88: 11-20, 1998.

[6] Eichler, AF, Loeffler, JS. Multidisciplinary management of brain metastasis. Oncologist 12: 884-98, 2007.

[7] Smit and Marshall. Editorial, Community Oncology, 9: 250-258, 2012.

[8] Villano, JL, Seery, TE, Bressler, LR. Temozolomide in malignant gliomas: current use and future targets. Cancer Chemotherapy and Pharmacology, 64: 647-655, 2009.

[9] Thompson, JA. Ten years of progress in melanoma. JNCCN, 10: 931-35, 2012.

[10] Genomics and Personalized Medicine Act of 2006; Bill of Congress 1093822.

[11] Wollemann, M. Biochemistry of brain tumours, University Park Press, Baltimore, 1974.

[12] Warburg, O. The Metabolism of tumours, Constable, London, 1930.

[13] Szent-Gyorgyi, A. The Living State and Cancer, New York, NY, Marcel Dekker, Inc. 1978, pp. 21-24.

[14] Klotz, IM, Rosenberg, RM. Introduction to chemical thermodynamics, WA Benjamin, Inc, Menlo Park, CA, 1964.

[15] Wald, G. Life in the second and third periods; or why phosphorus and sulfur for high energy bonds? In: Horizons in Biochemistry, Ed. Kasha, M, Pullman, Academic Press, New York, 1962, pp.127-142.

[16] Morgan, LR, Struck, RF, Rodgers, AH, Bastian, G, Jursic, BS, Papaginnis, C, Waud, W. Intracerebral metabolism and pharmacokinetics of 4-demethyl-4-cholesteryl-oxy-carbonylpenclomedine (DM-CHOC-PEN). Proc. Amer. Assoc. Res., 49: Abst. 3745, 2008.

[17] Shealy YF, Krauth CA, Laster WR. 2-Chloroethylmethylsulfonyl)methanesulfonate and related (methylsulfonyl)methanesulfonates. Antineoplastic activity in vivo. J. Med. Chem. 27: 664-670, 1984; Dykes DJ, Waud WR, Harrison SD, Griswold DP, Shealy YF, Montgomery JA. Antitumor activity of 2-chloroethyl (ethylsulfonyl)meth-ane-sulfonate (clomesone, NSC 33847) against selected tumor systems in mice. Cancer Res. 49: 1182-1186, 1989.

[18] Klotz, IM. Energy changes in biochemical reactions, Academic Press, New York, 1967.

[19] Morgan, LR, Struck, RF, Waud, WR, LeBlanc, B, Rodgers, AH, Jursic, BS. Carbonate and carbamate derivatives of 4-demethylpenclomedine as novel anticancer agents. Cancer Chemotherapy and Pharmacology, 64: 829-836, 2009.

[20] Morgan, LR, Rodgers, AH, Bastian, G, Struck, RF, Waud, WR. Comparative pharma-cokinetics and intermediary metabolism of 4-demethyl-4-cholesteryl- oxycarbonyl-penclomedine (DM-CHOC-PEN), EORTC/AACR/NCI, 567, 2010.

[21] Morgan, LR, Struck, RF, Rodgers, AH, Serota, DG. Preclinical Toxicity of 4- Demeth-yl-4-cholestryloxyl-carbonylpenclomedine (DM-CHOC-PEN). Proc. Amer. Assoc. Res., 48: abst. 5614, 2007.

[22] Pletsas, D, Wheelhouse, RT, Pletsa, V, Nicolaou, A, Jenkins, TC, Bibby, MC, Kyto-poulas, SA. Polar, Functionalized guanine-O^6 derivatives resistant to repair by O^6-al-kylguanine-DNA alkyltransferase: implications for the design of DNA-modifying drugs, Eur. J. Med Chem., 11: 1-10, 2006.

[23] Morgan, LR. Demethylpenclomedine analogs and their use as anti-cancer agents. US Patent 8,124,596, 2012.

[24] Morgan, LR IND 0688876 DM-CHOC-PEN- Study May Proceed, FDA September 24, 2010.

[25] Weiner, RS, Friedlander, P, Gordon, C, Ware, ML, Bastian, G, Rodgers, AH, Urien, S, Morgan, LR. Comparative Pharmacokinetics of 4-Demethyl-4-cholesteryloxycarbo-nylpenclomedine (DM-CHOC-PEN) in Humans, Proc. Amer. Assoc. Cancer Res., 53: 758, 2012.

[26] Philip Friedlander, Personnel communication.

[27] Morgan, LR. Complexes of 4-hydroperoxyifosfamide as antitumor agents, EU Patent 107060956, 2012.

[28] Morgan, LR, Benes, E, Rodgers, AH, Jursic, BS, Struck, BF, Waud, WR, Weiner, RS, Ware, M, Friedlander, P. Interaction of 4-Demethyl-4-cholesteryloxycarbonyl penclo-medine (DM-CHOC-PEN) with Melanoma Melanin Metabolism and Cell Death, EC-CO, Abst. 457, 2011.

[29] Morgan, LR, Rodgers, AH, Bastian, G, Papagiannis, C, Krietlow, D, Struck, RF, Waud, WR. Comparative pharmacokinetics and intermediary metabolism of 4-de-methyl-4-cholesteryloxycarbonylpenclomedine (DM-CHOC-PEN), EORTC/AACR/NCI, Abstr. 458, 2010.

[30] Morgan, LR, Singh, R. Cytochrome oxidase-succinic dehydrogenase activities and the melanin pigment cycle in poikilothermic vertebrates. Comp. Biochem. Physiol., 28: 83-94, 1969.

[31] Morgan, LR, Singh, R, Sylvest, V, Weimort, D. Oxidation of o-phenols by mouse and human melanoma dihydroxyphenyl alanine oxidase and dihydroxyphenyl alanine. Cancer Res. 27: 2395-2407, 1967.

[32] Rapier, HS. The aerobic oxidation. Physiol. Revs. 245-288, 1928.

[33] Mason, HS. Structure of Melanins, In: Pigment Cell Biology, Ed. Gordon, M. Academic Press Inc, Publishers, New York, 1959, pp. 563-582.

[34] Van Woert, HH, Nicholson, A, Cotzias, GC. Functional similarities between the cyto-plasmic organelles of melanocytes and mitochondria of hepatocytes. Nature, 208, 810-811, 1965.

[35] Traub, EF, Spoor, HJ. Melanin and tyrosinase in skin pigmentation. In: Pigment Cell Growth, 3rd Conference on Biology of Normal and Atypical Pigment Cell Growth. Ed.: Myron Gordon, pp. 211-219, 1953, NYNY Academic Press.

[36] Pullmans, A and Pullman, B. The band structure of melanin. Biochem. Biophys. Acta, 54, 384-485, 1961.

[37] Zolwyski, M., and Baker, L.H. Ifosfamide. J. Natl. Cancer Inst. 80:556-566, 1988.

[38] Norpoth, K. Studies on the metabolism of isophosphamide in man. Cancer Treat. Rep. 60:437-443, 1976.

[39] Struck, RF, Dykes, DJ, Corbett, TH, Suling, WJ, MW. Isophosphoroamide mustard, a metabolite of ifosfamide with activity against murine tumors comparable to cyclophosphamide. Brit. J. Cancer 47:15-26, 1983.

[40] Goren, MP, Wright, RK, Pratt, CB, Pell, FE. Dechloroethylation of ifosfamide and neurotoxicity. Lancet 2:1219-1220, 1986.

[41] Cox, PJ. Cyclophosphamide cystitis – Identification of acrolein as the causativet. Biochem. Pharmacol. 28:2045-2049, 1979.

[42] Seo, IS, Clark, SA, McGovern, FD, Clark, DL, Johnson, EH. Leiomyosarcoma of the urinary bladder 13 years after cyclophosphamide therapy for Hodgkin's disease. Cancer 55:1597-1603, 1985.

[43] Colburn, KK, Cao, JD, Krick, EH, Mortensen, SE, Wong, LG. Hodgkins lymphoma in a patient treated for Wegeners granulomatosis with cyclophosphamide and azathioprine. J. Rheumatol. 12:599-602, 1985.

[44] Cuzick, J, Erskine, S, Edelman, D, Gelton, DAG. A comparison of the incidence of myelodyplastic syndrome and acute myeloid leukemia following melphalan and cyclophosphamide treatment for myelomatosis. Brit. J. Cancer 55:523-530, 1987.

[45] Durst, J., Ahrens, S., Paulussen, M., Rube, C., Winkelmann, W., Zoubek, A., Harms, D. and Jurgens, H. Second malignancies after treatment for Ewing's sarcoma: report of the CESS-studies. Int. J. Radiat. Oncol. Biol. Phys. 42:379-384, 1998.

[46] Narayanan, V. In vivo evaluation of 4-hydroperoxyifosfamide (NSC 207117 and 227114). Screening Data Summary, Dev. Ther. Program, Dir. Cancer Treat. NCI, Bethesda, MD 20205.

[47] Morgan, L.R, Struck, R.F. Rodgers, A.H., Jursic, B.S., Waud, W.S., Butera, D., Development of Clinical Products. NCI Translational Science Meeting, Washington, DC, 2008.

[48] Morgan, L.R., Struck, R.F., Rodgers, A.H., Jursic, B.S. Waud, W. R. Pre- clinical Pharmacology and Toxicology for 4-Hydeoperoxyifosfamide (HOOI) and its L-lysine Salt – A Novel Anticancer Agent. Amer. Assoc Cancer Res, 42, 3222, 2011; Cancer Chemotherapy Pharmacology, submitted.

[49] Morgan, LR, Benes, E, Rodgers, AH, Jursic, BS, Friedlander, P, Weiner, RS, Ware, ML, Struck, RF. 4-Demethyl-4-cholesterylcarbonylpenclomedine (DM-CHOC-PEN) and 4-Hydroperoxyifosfamide (HOOI) as Binary Therapy for Melanoma, EORTC/AACR/NCI, Abst, 703, 2011.

[50] Robert F. Struck, Personnel communication.

Chapter 2

DNA-PK is a Potential Molecular Therapeutic Target for Glioblastoma

P. O. Carminati, F. S. Donaires, P. R. D. V. Godoy,
A. P. Montaldi, J. A. Meador, A.S. Balajee,
G. A. Passos and E. T. Sakamoto-Hojo

Additional information is available at the end of the chapter

1. Introduction

Glioblastoma multiforme is one of the deadliest forms of brain tumor with a median survival of <12 months with a high rate of recurrence. Glioblastoma cells respond poorly to radiotherapy and chemotherapy due to elevated DNA repair efficiency coupled with anti-apoptotic mechanisms [1, 2]. Therefore, development of new therapeutic strategies is absolutely critical either to control or cure the disease. Since glioblastoma cells have inherently elevated levels of DNA damage response (DDR) and DNA repair efficiency, we sought to determine whether or not suppression of key DNA repair factor(s) might be effective in sensitizing the brain tumor cells to chemotherapy. To test our objective, a pair of isogenic glioblastoma cell lines that differ in the functional status of DNA dependent protein kinase (DNA-PK) has been chosen. DNA dependent protein kinase (DNA-PK) belongs to a super family of phosphatidylinositol-3 kinase like kinases (PIKK) which also includes the gene products of ataxia telangiectasia mutated (ATM) and ATM and Rad 3 related (ATR) kinases [3, 4]. DNA-PK is the main component of mammalian NHEJ (non-homologous end joining), and also plays a role as a sensor of DNA damage by phosphorylating several downstream targets [5]. Further, DNA-PK has been demonstrated to be an important component of nucleotide excision repair (NER) pathway, which is chiefly responsible for the repair of bulky and helix distorting lesions induced by ultraviolet radiation (UV) and chemotherapeutic drugs such as cisplatin. To determine whether or not DNA-PK is a potential molecular therapeutic target for glioblastoma, two agents with different modes of action have been chosen for our study: (1) Zebularine and (2) Cisplatin.

Many tumor cells have characteristic epigenetic alterations involving genome wide DNA hypo-methylation and gene specific hyper-methylation at CpG dinucleotide sequences leading to aberrant silencing of critical genes involved in DNA damage response, cell cycle and DNA metabolic processes. Recent studies [6-8] have demonstrated the usefulness of epigenetic targeting in treating many cancer cell types through inhibition of histone deacetylases (HDAC) or DNA methyl transferases (DNMTs). Zebularine is a potent inhibitor of DNMTs and is superior to 5-AzaCR in terms of lower cytotoxicity and increased stability in aqueous solutions [9]. While Zebularine is a DNA-demethylating agent, cisplatin is a DNA cross-linking agent that induces the formation of DNA inter- and intra-strand cross-links. These cross-links are removed preferentially by NER pathway and NER deficient tumor cells are often sensitized to cisplatin treatment. Since DNA-PK plays a critical role in genome surveillance and DNA repair mechanisms, we wished to evaluate the potential of DNA-PK as a molecular therapeutic target for glioblastoma.

2. DNA-PK deficient cells are sensitive to zebularine and cisplatin treatments

2.1. Zebularine sensitizes DNA–PK deficient glioblastoma cells

DNA-PK deficient (MO59J) and proficient (MO59K) glioblastoma cells were purchased from American Type Culture Collection (Rockville, MD, USA). Cells were routinely cultured in OPTI-MEM supplemented with 5% fetal bovine serum, vitamins and antibiotics. Zebularine [1-beta-D-ribofuranosyl]-1, 2-dihydropyrimidin-2-one] was purchased from EMD Biosciences (San Diego, CA, USA). Zebularine was dissolved in dimethyl sulfoxide (DMSO) at a stock concentration of 100 mM and stored at 4ºC. Clonogenic survival and proliferations assays were carried to determine the sensitivity of human gliomas (MO59J and MO59K) to different Zebularine concentrations (0-300 µM). The LC50 value for Zebularine was found to be 245 µM for DNA-PK deficient MO59J cells and at this concentration the survival of MO59K cells was reduced only by 20% [10]. This finding indicates that lack of DNA-PK potentiates the sensitization of gliomas to Zebularine. In contrast to MO59K cells, DNA-PK deficient cells (MO59J) showed a reduction in survival (20%) even at the lowest Zebularine concentration (10 µM). Further, an elevated frequency of polyploid cells observed specifically in MO59J cells after Zebularine treatment pointed out a mitotic checkpoint deficiency. Although depletion of DNMT1 by Zebularine occurred at similar levels in both glioblastoma cell lines, DNA-PK deficient MO59J cells displayed elevated DNA hypo-methylation detected both at genome overall and gene promoter levels. Consistent with increased sensitivity, deoxy-Zebularine adduct level, measured for the first time by us in the genomic DNA, was 3-6 fold higher in DNA-PK deficient MO59J cells relative MO59K cells. Elevated micronuclei frequency was also observed in MO59J cells indicating the impairment of DNA damage response and repair. Collectively, our study suggests that DNA-PK is a potentially useful molecular therapeutic target for gliomas.

2.2. DNA–PK deficient cells are sensitive to cisplatin treatment

The relationship between DNA-PK/Ku activity and cisplatin sensitivity has been observed earlier in gliomas. Gliomas with high expression level of DNA-PK are resistant to cisplatin [11]. In an earlier review, we suggested that DNA-PK inhibition may be a promising strategy for treating glioblastomas [for review see 12]. To determine the role of DNA-PK in conferring cisplatin resistance, MO59J and MO59K cells were treated with cisplatin (5-75 µM; Sigma Aldrich, USA) for 72 h and assayed for proliferation using a fluorescence based CyQuant assay (Invitrogen, USA). MO59J showed a greater sensitivity to cisplatin compared to MO59K, and displayed a dose dependent decrease in cell proliferation, being reduced to 20% relative to the vehicle (DMSO) treated control cells for the highest drug concentration (75 µM). In contrast, MO59K was sensitive to cisplatin only at high doses (>50 µM). These results clearly indicate that DNA-PK is a critical factor for cellular protection against cisplatin (Figure 1).

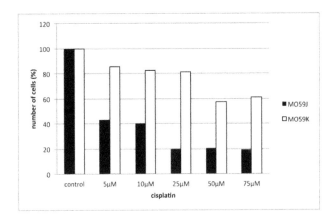

Figure 1. Cell proliferation assay using CyQuant (Invitrogen, USA) in MO59K and MO59J cells treated with cisplatin (5, 10, 25, 50, and 75 µM) for 72 h.

Cell cycle analysis was next performed to verify whether the enhanced cisplatin cytotoxicity of MO59J cells was due to defective cell cycle checkpoints. MO59K and MO59J cells in exponential growth phase were exposed to different concentrations (5 to 25 µM) of cisplatin and the cell cycle profile was analyzed by flow cytometry (24, 48 and 72 h after treatment). While DNA-PK proficient MO59K cells displayed an efficient accumulation of S-phase cells at all the concentrations of cisplatin exposure up to 72 h (Figure 2A), DNA-PK mutant MO59J cells exhibited only a modest S-phase accumulation after 24 h of drug treatment (25 µM cisplatin) (Figure 2B), which was alleviated at later time points (48 and 72 h).

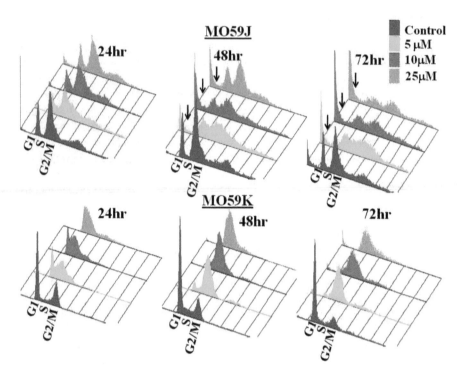

Figure 2. Cell cycle analysis for MO59K and MO59J cells treated with 5, 10 and 25 μM of cisplatin for 24, 48 and 72 h. DMSO was used as control.

Consistent with impaired cell cycle regulation, an increased frequency of apoptosis (43% for 25 μM cisplatin) was observed after cisplatin treatment in MO59J cells; in contrast to MO59K, DNA-PK deficient MO59J cells showed apoptotic death even at 5 μM of cisplatin (Figure 3A,B).

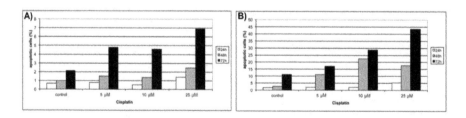

Figure 3. Frequency of apoptotic MO59K (A) and MO59J (B) cells detected by flow cytometry as a subG1 population after exposure to different concentrations of cisplatin (5, 10 and 25 μM). The results were obtained at 24, 48 and 72 h after treatment. 10,000 events were analyzed for each experiment.

Proliferating cell nuclear antigen (PCNA) is recruited to chromatin rapidly after DNA damage and the kinetics of disassembly from the chromatin is considered to reflect the DNA repair efficiency [13, 14]. PCNA expression was evaluated by Western blot in cisplatin- treated MO59K and MO59J cells. The expression of PCNA was increased in a dose-dependent manner in MO59K cells after 24 h of drug treatment, while a constant level of PCNA expression was observed in MO59J cells indicating the lack of S-phase specific PCNA accumulation (Figure 4). Our results from MO59K and MO59J cell lines indicate that DNA-PK is a critical determinant of cell survival after cisplatin treatment and the lack of S-phase arrest (as seen in MO59J cells) is presumably responsible for the increased cell death after drug treatment.

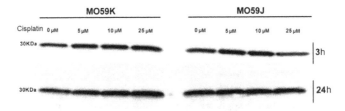

Figure 4. Expression of PCNA protein (30 KDa) analyzed by Western blot using specific antibody. MO59K and MO59J cells were treated with 5, 10 and 25 μM of cisplatin for 3 and 24 h. β-actin was used as control.

Therefore, DNA-PK may be an important molecule conferring cisplatin resistance in glioblastoma cells, with potential use as a molecular target, and we also observed that the combined effect of cisplatin and LY294002 (an inhibitor of DNA-PK) caused a significant decrease in cell proliferation and an increase in apoptotic cell death in glioma cell lines [15]. Our studies thus far performed indicate that the specific targeting of DNA-PK by small molecule inhibitors may be an effective strategy for the treatment of gliomas.

3. *In silico* analysis of transcription factors associated with differentially expressed genes in GBM cells

3.1. Introduction

Transcription factors (TFs) regulate gene expression by binding to specific DNA sequences of gene promoter regions. Their expression can be deregulated under certain pathological conditions, such as cancer. Therefore, studies on regulatory elements of the transcription machinery are essential for understanding the mechanisms involved in the regulation of oncogenes and tumor suppressor genes. Additionally, knowledge of the essential functions of TFs, may lead to strategic development of novel chemotherapy regimen for selectively killing cancer cells.

TFs play a critical role in various cellular processes through regulation of genes involved in cell cycle, proliferation, cell differentiation, and apoptosis. It has been suggested that TFs can be potential therapeutic targets for treating the patients with prostate [16] and breast cancer [17]. Recently, *in silico* prediction for regulation of TFs has been effectively utilized for diagnostics and therapeutics of breast cancer [17]. Identification and characterization of activated transcription regulatory elements hold a great promise not only in providing information on neoplastic mechanisms, but also in predicting targets for therapeutic intervention [18]. Although enormous amount of data exist for genes that are differentially expressed in tumor cells, knowledge of TFs associated with these genes is rather limited. Information on TFs may enable us to understand how differentially expressed genes in tumor cells respond to anticancer drugs, as a single or combined treatment with DNA repair inhibitors, which targets DNA repair proteins.

DNA-PK, one of the key components of mammalian NHEJ (non-homologous end joining) repair process, belongs to PI3K-related protein kinase (PIKK) family [19]. Recent studies have projected DNA-PK as a potential molecular target for cancer treatment. Many known PI3K inhibitors such as LY294002, wortmannin and PI-103, inhibit DNA-PK activity with a comparable potency to that observed for PI3K inhibition [20]. LY294002 is a PI3K (phosphatidylinositol-3 kinase) inhibitor, well recognized by its antitumor and pro-apoptotic properties in several cancer cell lines [21]. Although LY294002 alone can inhibit cell proliferation or induce apoptosis in cancer cells, its cytotoxic effects can be further enhanced when combined with radio- or chemotherapy [12, 22]. Consequently, PI3K inhibitors including LY294002 have been investigated as a possible adjuvant for cancer therapy in many tumor models [23-25], and its synergistic effects with other anti-tumoral drugs deserve to be investigated in cancer cells.

Our recent study demonstrated that a combined treatment of cisplatin (5-50µM) and LY294002 (50µM) for 24 h reduced the survival of U343 GBM cells with elevated apoptotic death at 72 h [15]. In this study, gene expression analysis was also performed using a glass slide microarray containing 4,300 cDNA clones from the human IMAGE Consortium cDNA library [http://image.llnl.gov/image/] essentially following the procedures published earlier [26]. Statistical analysis of the results [27] showed that 25µM cisplatin alone caused significant changes in the expression of 108 genes (28 up- and 80 down-regulated), while LY294002 alone altered the expression of 33 genes (6 up- and 27 down-regulated); additionally, 274 genes (97 up- and 177 down-regulated) were modulated by the combined treatment of cisplatin and LY294002. The complete gene lists are available at http//www.rge.fmrp.usp.br/passos/cislygbm/. The drug combination induced 2.6-fold higher numbers of modulated genes, relative to cisplatin alone, and these genes participate in several biological processes, such as DNA repair, cell death, and cell cycle control/proliferation, metabolism, transcription regulation, and cellular adhesion.

Using the gene sets obtained in the above-mentioned study, we performed an *in silico* analysis of TFs for the differentially expressed genes obtained in the following comparisons: 25µM cisplatin *versus* control, and 25µM cisplatin plus 50µM LY294002 *versus* control; these lists contained 108 and 274 differentially expressed genes (SAM analysis, FDR ≤ 0.05), respectively. Among the 274 genes, 97 (35.4%) genes were up-regulated and 177 (64.6%) genes were down-regulated. Both up- and down-regulated genes were submitted separately to *in silico* analysis through the FatiGO tool, Babelomics v3.2 [28]. For comparisons, the entire list of genes present in the microarray was subjected to analysis (4,300 transcripts).The data were analyzed by the two-tailed Fisher's exact test, with significance threshold for the p-values set at 0.05. Similar procedures were performed for the list of 108 genes (set of differentially expressed genes under 25μM cisplatin treatment). Information regarding the biological functions was obtained at SOURCE (http://smd.stanford.edu/cgi-bin/source/sourceSearch), and NCBI AceView (http://www.ncbi.nlm.nih.gov/IEB/Research/Acembly/).

3.2. TFs associated with up–regulated genes

Among the predicted TFs associated with up-regulated genes after treatment with cisplatin alone, the most significant ones are AHR (p = 9.9E–3, 7.7% of associated genes), HNF4 (p = 9.6E–3, 81% of associated genes), NFkappaB (p = 5.8E–3, 11.5% of associated genes), MRF2 (p = 1.9E–3, 53.8%), and SOX5 (p = 1.6E–2, 7.7% of associated genes). These TFs have been linked with distinct biological functions, including differentiation, homeostasis, cell growth, senescence and apoptosis. AHR regulates an array of physiological responses including xenobiotic metabolism, vasculature development, immunosuppression, T-cell differentiation, reproduction, and cell cycle progression [29]. Most genes known to be controlled by HNF4α are involved in lipid, carbohydrate or amino acid transport and metabolism, indicating a central role in energy homeostasis [30]. MRF2 (ARID5B) plays a vital role in regulating embryonic development, cell growth and differentiation through tissue-specific repression of differentiation-specific gene expression [31, 32]. Aberrant *ARID5B* expression in developing fetus could halt B-lymphocyte maturation and contribute to leukemogenesis [33]. SOX5 is involved in gene regulation and maintenance of chromatin structure during diverse developmental processes. Recently, SOX5 has been found associated with induced acute cellular senescence [34], while NFkappaB is related to apoptosis evasion in GBM cells [35, 36].

Term	Percentage with term		Enrichment index	p-value
	List #1	List #2		
GATA-3	30.1	16.3	1.85	1.7E–3
FOXP3	60.2	46.0	1.31	8.0E–3
FOXJ2	46.2	32.6	1.42	9.5E–3
C/EBP	18.3	9.8	1.87	1.5E–2
LXR, PXR, CAR COUP, RAR	62.4	54.6	1.14	1.6E–2

Table 1. Transcription factors (Term) associated with up-regulated genes in cisplatin and LY294002 treated U343 cells. "Percentage with term" corresponds to the amount of genes that was associated to each TF in each list: List #1 represents up-regulated genes obtained by statistical analysis, and List #2 represents all the genes present in the microarray slide. "Enrichment index" was calculated for each Term by dividing the percentage in the List #1 by that in the List #2.

For the combined treatment (cisplatin and LY294002), the predicted TFs associated with up-regulated genes showed different TFs (Table 1), indicating that the drug combination induced quantitative and qualitative differences in transcript expression profiles displayed by GBM treated cells.

All the TFs that were associated with up-regulated genes showed enrichment indexes greater than 1 (in the range of 1.14 to 1.87), indicating that these TFs were more specifically associated with the up-regulated genes as compared to the entire array of genes (Table 1). Biological functions of the predicted TFs associated with up- and down-regulated genes after the combined treatment (cisplatin and LY294002) in U343 cells are described below:

GATA-3 (*Trans-acting T-cell-specific transcription factor*) gene encodes a protein, which belongs to the GATA family of transcription factors. The protein contains two GATA-type zinc fingers and is an important regulator of T-cell development and plays an important role in endothelial cell biology; GATA-3 is essential in the embryonic development of the parathyroid, auditory system and kidneys, and defects in this gene cause HDR syndrome (hypoparathyroidism with sensorineural deafness and renal dysplasia) [37]. GATA-3 analysis and the phenotypic spectrum obtained for nine Japanese families with the HDR syndrome suggest that this syndrome is primarily caused by GATA-3 haploinsufficiency [38]. This TF plays a dual role in transcription regulation in a positive and negative manner. In accordance with this, we found the association of GATA-3 with up-regulated genes (EI = 1.85) after drug treatment in U343 cells.

Another TF, FOXP3 (*Forkhead box P3*), a positive regulator of transcription, plays a critical role in the control of immune response. This TF was associated with up-regulated genes (EI = 1.31) in drug-treated U343 cells. Defects in this gene lead to X-linked autoimmunity-immunodeficiency syndrome [39]. In several neoplasias, such as breast [40], ovarian [41], skin [42] and stomach, FOXP3 was found over-expressed [43], or mutated in prostate cancer [44]. It is well established that tumor cells acquire molecular and biochemical changes which make them potentially vulnerable to the immune system [45]. Alterations in the immune system can be applied for cancer detection and therapies [46]. Interestingly, [47] demonstrated a dependency on functional TP53 for DNA damage induced activation of *FOXP3* in human breast and colon carcinoma cells. However, the precise role of *FOXP3* in drug responses is still unknown.

FOXJ2 (*Forkhead box J2*) was also associated with up-regulated genes (EI = 1.42); this TF is often described as a positive regulator of transcription [48] and is a member of Forkhead Box TFs, many of which have been reported to participate in tumor migration and invasion. Wang et al. [49] showed that the expression of *FOXJ2* was high in primary breast cancer tissues without lymph nodes metastases; moreover, *FOXJ2* may play a role in maintenance and survival of developing and adult neurons, but its function in the central nervous system is still unclear. Knockdown of this TF in cultured primary astrocytes by siRNA showed that *FOXJ2* played an important role in lipopolysaccharide-induced inflammatory responses [50]. Nonetheless, there is no information in the literature about its function in relation to chemotherapeutic drugs.

C/EBP (*CCAAT/enhancer-binding protein*) family plays important roles in many processes such as cell differentiation, metabolism, and development. *C/EBP* (CEBPA) gene, CCAAT/enhancer binding protein alpha, involved in cell cycle arrest [51], and also plays a role in DNA damage response dependent on TP53 [52]. The protein acts as a dominant-negative inhibitor by forming hetero-dimers with other C/EBP members, such as C/EBP and LAP (*liver activator protein*), and preventing their DNA binding activity. Another member, GADD153 (CHOP), is a critical initiator of ER stress-induced apoptosis, and its knockdown prevents perturbations in the *AKT* (*protein kinase B*)/*FOXO3a* (*forkhead box, class O, 3a*) pathway in response to ER stress [53]. C/EBP β, a member of a subfamily of basic leucine zipper (bZIP) protein family, play a potential role in the proliferation and invasion of glioma, being considered as a novel molecular target for therapy, as well as a predictive marker for survival of patients with glioma [54]. In the present study, C/EBP showed an association with up-regulated genes (EI = 1.87), suggesting a possible role in DNA damage responses under drug treatment, and most probably, via AKT pathway, which is a target for LY294002.

Three TFs (*LXR*, *PXR* and *CAR*) were related to the same percentage (62.4%) of up-regulated genes, presenting EI = 1.14. The *liver X receptors* (*LXR*), *LXRA* and *LXRB*, comprise a subfamily of the nuclear receptor superfamily and are key regulators of macrophage function, controlling transcriptional programs involved in lipid homeostasis and inflammation. Polymorphism of *LXR* gene is associated with obesity since this gene is involved in cellular lipid metabolic process [55]. *PXR*, also named *NR1I2* (*Nuclear receptor subfamily 1, group I, member 2*) is a TF that acts in both positive and negative regulation of transcription, as well as in xenobiotic transport and metabolic process, in addition to exogenous drug catabolic process; this gene seems to be also implicated in breast cancer development [56, 57]. Similarly to *PXR*, *CAR* (*NR1I3, Nuclear receptor subfamily 1, group I, member 3*) is also a key regulator of xenobiotic and endobiotic metabolism [58]. Identification of TFs related to liver and xenobiotic metabolism regulating the over-expressed genes suggests that these genes may play a role in drug responses. However, this interesting possibility needs further validation.

The foregoing account demonstrates that all the TFs that are associated with up-regulated genes after combined treatment (cisplatin and LY294002) are regulators of important biological processes, such as cell differentiation, metabolism, development, and immune response, but the literature is still scarce regarding the role of above mentioned TFs in cellular response mechanisms to chemotherapeutic drugs. In spite of this, the increment observed in the number of associated genes (in terms of EI index, which ranged from 1.14 to 1.87) tends to suggest the involvement of these TFs in the outcome of cellular response to combined treatment.

3.3. TFs associated with down–regulated genes

Similar to the prediction of TFs associated with up-regulated genes, we performed the same kind of analysis for determining the TFs associated with down-regulated genes. None of the TF was found associated with down-regulated genes after treatment with cisplatin alone. However, for the combined treatment (cisplatin and LY294002), six TFs were predicted (Table 2). All TFs displayed enrichment indexes greater than 1 (ranging from 1.10 to 1.80), indicating that the enrichment was greater in the list of down-regulated genes (list #1) in comparison to all the genes (list #2) included in the array.

Term	Percentage with term		Enrichment index	p-value
	List #1	List #2		
GATA-3	23.6	16.3	1.45	2.2E–2
Evi-1	50	38.1	1.31	3.9E–2
HNF-1	90.2	84.0	1.10	4.8E–2
USF1	26.4	20.1	1.31	5.1E–2
CDX	82.2	67.3	1.22	5.6E–2
AP-1	27.6	15.5	1.80	5.6E–2

Table 2. Transcription factors (Term) associated to down-regulated genes in treated U343 cells (cisplatin combined to LY294002) vs. control. "Percentage with term" corresponds to the amount of genes that was associated to each TF in each list: list #1 represents the down-regulated genes obtained in the statistical analysis, and list #2 represents all genes present in the microarray slide. An "Enrichment index" was calculated for each Term by dividing the percentage in the list #1 by that in the list #2.

GATA-3, as already described above, was found associated with both up- and down-regulated genes. This could be due to the dual activity of this TF, which acts as a positive or negative regulator of transcription. GATA-3 also participates in the negative regulation of cell proliferation process, which can be triggered as a response to drug treatments. Accordingly, we found GATA-3 association with down-regulated genes (EI = 1.45) after drug treatment in U343 cells.

EVI-1, also known as *RUNX1* (*Runt-related transcription factor 1*), is a positive regulator of transcription related to peripheral nervous system, neuron development, hematopoietic stem cell proliferation, and angiogenesis, among other functions. Due to its role in hematopoietic and nervous systems, deregulation of this TF results in hematological disorders [59-62] and central nervous system diseases [63]. Recently, Satoh et al. [64] reported that the C-terminal deletion of RUNX1 attenuates DNA-damage repair responses in hematopoietic stem/progenitor cells, and additionally, they found that *RUNX1* directly regulates the transcription of *GADD45A* gene, which is involved in cell cycle arrest. Association of EVI-1 with down-regulated genes (EI = 1.31) presumably indicates an impaired function of this TF in U343 cells, since it is expected to positively regulate the gene targets.

HNF-1 is also named *HNF1A* (*Hepatocyte Nuclear Factor 1 Alpha*) and *TCF-1* (*Transcription Factor 1*). This TF, previously related to diseases such as diabetes and neoplasias [65-70], encodes a protein involved in the WNT signaling pathway [71]. The activation of this pathway has been pointed as one of the main causes of colon cancer; in addition, it has been reported that *HNF1A* plays an important role in transduction of this pathway in the intestine [72]. Furthermore, Roth et al. [73] demonstrated alterations in the regulation of WNT signaling pathway in glioma cells. Inhibition of genes participating in the WNT pathway promote blockage of tumor growth [74].This is compatible with reduction in cell survival after drug treatment in GBM cells which may be most likely due to down-regulation of several genes regulated by *HNF1A*.

USF1 (*Upstream transcription factor 1*), another TF predicted in our analysis, is a gene with known functions in cellular responses under stress conditions, such as UV and hypoxia. In breast tumors, a role for *USF1* in regulating the expression of *estrogen receptor alpha* (*ERalpha*) has been demonstrated [75]. Recently, Baron et al. [76] demonstrated a role for USF-1 in maintaining genome integrity in response to UV-induced DNA photolesions. Additionally, using a mouse knock out model, the authors showed that the loss of USF-1 compromises DNA repair, suggesting that USF-1 may play a similar role in human cells. However, in the present study, USF1 was found associated with down-regulated genes (EI = 1.31) in U343 and the role of USF1 remains to be investigated in tumor cells.

CDX represents a gene family of *caudal-related homeobox* TFs, composed of the following members: *CDX1*, *CDX2*, and *CDX4*. All these members participate in the regulation of intestine-specific gene expression, and also in anterior-posterior pattern specification and blood vessel development. These TFs have been found associated with several neoplasias, including esophageal [77, 78], gallbladder [79], liver [80], colorectal [81-83], and pancreatic [84], but their role in drug responses is still unknown.

AP-1 (presented EI = 1.8) is a TF complex formed by proteins of the JUN family dimerized with members of the *FOS* gene family, which consists of 4 members (*FOS*, *FOSB*, *FOSL1*, and *FOSL2*) that encode leucine zipper proteins. All these genes are oncogenes with established roles in neoplastic cell transformation [85-87], prostatic [88], colorectal [89, 90], liver [91, 92], stomach [93], and breast cancers [94]. Interestingly, Hamdi et al. [95] demonstrated the roles of AP-1 components, ATF3 and FRA1 (FOSL1), in JNK- and ERK-dependent cell cycle arrest and apoptosis after cisplatin or UV-light treatments, by activating both JNK and ERK pathways in human glioblastoma cells lacking functional TP53. Recently, Meise et al. [96] showed that *FOSL1* (*FRA1*) was up-regulated in glioblastoma cells following nimustine (ACNU) treatment. Thus, it becomes apparent that the AP-1 complex also participates in drug responses, and could be activated by combined treatment of cisplatin and LY294002 in GBM cells.

Therefore, TFs associated with down-regulated genes are critical participants in several biological processes such as neuron development, WNT signaling pathway, cellular response under stress conditions, and neoplastic cell transformation. It seems that all these TFs work in a concerted manner to regulate several genes leading to initiation of cellular responses after the combined treatment of cisplatin and LY294002 in GBM cells. Since most of the TFs predicted by us were not included in the gene arrays, expression of these TFS after drug treatment could not be verified. Further experiments are certainly warranted to understand their concerted roles in understanding the cellular response mechanisms to cisplatin and LY294002.

TFs and cis-regulatory elements are considered key components for transcription regulation [97]. Specific TFs can be involved in the control of co-expressed genes [98], and these genes tend to participate in related pathways, for example, cell cycle control and apoptosis [99, 100]. Thus, search for the common TFs that control the transcription of a specific group of genes such as those involved in DNA repair or replication may provide biomarkers, which can be potential targets for therapeutic intervention [101]. Interestingly, some of the predicted TFs were recently reported to be associated with DNA repair/DNA damage responses in human cells, but few were reported in GBM. Nevertheless, the TFs predicted by *in silico* analysis described above may be useful for understanding how the transcription machinery responds to chemotherapeutic agents in GBM cells. Further studies are required to get insights regarding the role of TFs identified by us in modulating the drug response of GBM cells.

3.4. Signaling pathways involved in drug responses

In addition, data obtained on differentially expressed genes between treated (cisplatin combined to LY294002) and control U343 cells were submitted to a pathway analysis, using tools available in the Database for Annotation, Visualization and Integrated Discovery (DAVID) v6.7 [102]. The KEGG pathway analysis was selected and pathways presenting p-values $\leq$ 0.05 were chosen.

Signaling pathway analysis was performed by means of tools available in DAVID, as previously described. This analysis allowed the identification of common biological pathways mapped in the KEGG pathway database, in which the up-regulated genes in treated U343 cells are involved. Three pathways were significantly associated with up regulated genes (Table 3), among which two are related to the inositol molecule (inositol phosphate metabolism and phosphatidylinositol signaling system); three genes (PIK3C3, PIP5K1B, OCRL) were included as participants of both pathways. The TP53 signaling pathway was also associated which included three important genes: ATR, CCNG1 and SESN1. These results are consistent with earlier studies demonstrating the activation of these signaling pathways under drug treatments [103-105].

KEGG term	Genes*	p-value
hsa00562: Inositol phosphate metabolism	PIK3C3, PIP5K1B, OCRL	3.3E-2
hsa04115: TP53 signaling pathway	ATR, CCNG1, SESN1	5.0E-2
hsa04070: Phosphatidylinositol signaling system	PIK3C3, PIP5K1B, OCRL	5.0E-2

* Genes participating in each pathway

Table 3. Cellular signaling pathways associated with up-regulated genes in treated U343 cells (cisplatin combined to LY294002), as analyzed by tools available in DAVID.

The PIK3C3 gene (Phosphoinositide-3-kinase, class 3) participates in the innate immune response and cell cycle. This gene also plays an essential role in regulating functional autophagy and is crucial for normal liver and heart function [106]. PIP5K1B (Phosphatidylinositol-4-phosphate 5-kinase, type I, beta) is involved in the biosynthesis of phosphatidylinositol 4,5-bisphosphate. The OCRL gene (Oculocerebrorenal syndrome of Lowe) encodes a phosphatase enzyme with a demonstrated role in actin polymerization, and it is an important participant in the trans-Golgi network. Mutations in this gene cause oculocerebrorenal syndrome of Lowe and also Dent disease [107].

The protein encoded by the ATR gene (Ataxia telangiectasia and Rad3 related) act in the cell cycle checkpoint and is required for cell cycle arrest and DNA damage repair in response to DNA damage. The ATR gene belongs to the PI3/PI4-kinase family, as well as ATM and DNA-PK, and is known as playing an important role in cellular response to cisplatin [108-110]. The aberrantly activated antiapoptotic phospatidyl-3-inositol-kinase (PI3K)/Akt signaling is induced by cisplatin and restricts the efficiency of chemotherapy [49]. The *CCNG1* gene (*cyclin G1*) plays a role in cell cycle and growth, brain development and G2/M checkpoint, acting in the negative regulation of apoptotic process. Altered regulation of this gene was observed in breast cancer [111], and leukemia [112]. *SESN1* (*Sestrin 1*) is responsible for the negative regulation of cell proliferation, acting in cell cycle arrest in response to DNA damage stimulus. This gene was found differentially induced by genotoxic stress (UV, gamma-irradiation and cytotoxic drugs) in a TP53-dependent manner, presenting properties common to the GADD family of growth arrest and DNA damage-inducible stress-response genes [113].

Therefore, we found relevant pathways related to TP53 (cell cycle arrest and DNA repair) in response to DNA damage, as well as to the inositol phosphate metabolism and signaling. Furthermore, several predicted TFs associated with modulated genes participate in "basal vital processes", and these processes include the inositol metabolism and signaling, highlighting the importance of these pathways in cellular response mechanisms after drug treatment. However, it is not known whether the observed sensitivity of GBM to cisplatin and LY294002 is due to disruption of some of the above-mentioned vital processes through inhibition of PI3K dependent signaling pathways. A likely possibility that needs consideration is that several sub-pathways can be inactivated/activated due to loss of major tumor suppressor genes such as PTEN, which negatively regulates PI3K/AKT pathways [114] in TP53 proficient U343 GBM cell line. [115]. Furthermore, TP53 pathway, which has been extensively studied in cancer, was also involved in U343 cell line after drug exposure.

3.5. Conclusion

Identification of TFs associated with a set of differentially expressed genes is an interesting approach that may allow to interpret mechanisms triggered in a cellular milieu after a given treatment condition. In the context of cancer research, differential expression of genes and pathways in response to drug treatment may either result in tumor growth reduction or cell killing.

Beside the relevance of our findings, some methodological limitations should be mentioned regarding *in silico* prediction of TFs. Numerous TF binding sites exist for each of the gene targets and it is hard to predict which binding site is critical for transcriptional regulation. It is possible that a considerable fraction of these binding sites are nonfunctional and may constitute biological noise [116]. Other choices, such as ChIP experiments, may overcome this concern by detecting indirect TF-DNA interactions through protein/protein interaction [117]. Even though most of the predicted TFs we identified in our study have not been specifically shown to be associated with GBM in previous studies, they can be considered as potential predictors for evaluating the effectiveness of drug response in GBM. Further verification and validation of the TFs involved in GBM may provide useful information for developing novel therapeutic strategies for brain tumors.

Author details

P. O. Carminati[1], F. S. Donaires[1], P. R. D. V. Godoy[1], A. P. Montaldi[1], J. A. Meador[2], A.S. Balajee[2], G. A. Passos[3] and E. T. Sakamoto-Hojo[1,4]

1 Department of Genetics, Faculty of Medicine of Ribeirão Preto, São Paulo University (USP), Ribeirão Preto, SP, Brazil

2 Center for Radiological Research, Department of Radiation Oncology, College of Physicians and Surgeons, Columbia University, New York, NY, USA

3 Department of Genetics, Faculty of Medicine and Faculty of Dentistry, University of São Paulo, Ribeirão Preto, SP, Brazil.

4 Department of Biology, Faculty of Philosophy, Sciences and Letters of Ribeirão Preto, São Paulo University (USP), Ribeirão Preto, SP, Brazil

References

[1] Bao, S, Q Wu, RE McLendon, et al., Glioma stem cells promote radioresistance by preferential activation of the DNA damage response. Nature, 2006. 444(7120): p. 756-60.

[2] Johannessen, TC, R Bjerkvig, and BB Tysnes, DNA repair and cancer stem-like cells-- potential partners in glioma drug resistance? Cancer Treat Rev, 2008. 34(6): p. 558-67.

[3] Durocher, D and SP Jackson, DNA-PK, ATM and ATR as sensors of DNA damage: variations on a theme? Curr Opin Cell Biol, 2001. 13(2): p. 225-31.

[4] Falck, J, J Coates, and SP Jackson, Conserved modes of recruitment of ATM, ATR and DNA-PKcs to sites of DNA damage. Nature, 2005. 434(7033): p. 605-11.

[5] Collis, SJ, TL DeWeese, PA Jeggo, et al., The life and death of DNA-PK. Oncogene, 2005. 24(6): p. 949-61.

[6] Jones, PA and SB Baylin, The fundamental role of epigenetic events in cancer. Nat Rev Genet, 2002. 3(6): p. 415-28.

[7] Jones, PA and SB Baylin, The epigenomics of cancer. Cell, 2007. 128(4): p. 683-92.

[8] Karagiannis, TC and A El-Osta, Clinical potential of histone deacetylase inhibitors as stand alone therapeutics and in combination with other chemotherapeutics or radiotherapy for cancer. Epigenetics, 2006. 1(3): p. 121-6.

[9] Cheng, JC, DJ Weisenberger, FA Gonzales, et al., Continuous zebularine treatment effectively sustains demethylation in human bladder cancer cells. Mol Cell Biol, 2004. 24(3): p. 1270-8.

[10] Meador, JA, Y Su, JL Ravanat, et al., DNA-dependent protein kinase (DNA-PK)-deficient human glioblastoma cells are preferentially sensitized by Zebularine. Carcinogenesis, 2010. 31(2): p. 184-91.

[11] Shao, CJ, J Fu, HL Shi, et al., Activities of DNA-PK and Ku86, but not Ku70, may predict sensitivity to cisplatin in human gliomas. J Neurooncol, 2008. 89(1): p. 27-35.

[12] Sakamoto-Hojo, ET and AS Balajee, Targeting poly (ADP) ribose polymerase I (PARP-1) and PARP-1 interacting proteins for cancer treatment. Anticancer Agents Med Chem, 2008. 8(4): p. 402-16.

[13] Balajee, AS, I Dianova, and VA Bohr, Oxidative damage-induced PCNA complex formation is efficient in xeroderma pigmentosum group A but reduced in Cockayne syndrome group B cells. Nucleic Acids Res, 1999. 27(22): p. 4476-82.

[14] Balajee, AS and CR Geard, Chromatin-bound PCNA complex formation triggered by DNA damage occurs independent of the ATM gene product in human cells. Nucleic Acids Res, 2001. 29(6): p. 1341-51.

[15] Carminati, PO, FS Donaires, MM Marques, et al., Cisplatin associated with LY294002 increases cytotoxicity and induces changes in transcript profiles of glioblastoma cells. manuscript in preparation, 2012.

[16] Sankpal, UT, S Goodison, M Abdelrahim, et al., Targeting Sp1 transcription factors in prostate cancer therapy. Med Chem, 2011. 7(5): p. 518-25.

[17] Liu, LY, LY Chang, WH Kuo, et al., In Silico Prediction for Regulation of Transcription Factors onTheir Shared Target Genes Indicates Relevant Clinical Implications in a Breast Cancer Population. Cancer Inform, 2012. 11: p. 113-37.

[18] Rhodes, DR, S Kalyana-Sundaram, V Mahavisno, et al., Mining for regulatory programs in the cancer transcriptome. Nat Genet, 2005. 37(6): p. 579-83.

[19] Anderson, CW and SP Lees-Miller, The nuclear serine/threonine protein kinase DNA-PK. Crit Rev Eukaryot Gene Expr, 1992. 2(4): p. 283-314.

[20] Kong, D, S Yaguchi, and T Yamori, Effect of ZSTK474, a novel phosphatidylinositol 3-kinase inhibitor, on DNA-dependent protein kinase. Biol Pharm Bull, 2009. 32(2): p. 297-300.

[21] Yamaguchi, K, SH Lee, JS Kim, et al., Activating transcription factor 3 and early growth response 1 are the novel targets of LY294002 in a phosphatidylinositol 3-kinase-independent pathway. Cancer Res, 2006. 66(4): p. 2376-84.

[22] Ohta, T, M Ohmichi, T Hayasaka, et al., Inhibition of phosphatidylinositol 3-kinase increases efficacy of cisplatin in in vivo ovarian cancer models. Endocrinology, 2006. 147(4): p. 1761-9.

[23] Kong, D and T Yamori, Phosphatidylinositol 3-kinase inhibitors: promising drug candidates for cancer therapy. Cancer Sci, 2008. 99(9): p. 1734-40.

[24] Prevo, R, E Deutsch, O Sampson, et al., Class I PI3 kinase inhibition by the pyridinyl-furanopyrimidine inhibitor PI-103 enhances tumor radiosensitivity. Cancer Res, 2008. 68(14): p. 5915-23.

[25] Westhoff, MA, JA Kandenwein, S Karl, et al., The pyridinylfuranopyrimidine inhibitor, PI-103, chemosensitizes glioblastoma cells for apoptosis by inhibiting DNA repair. Oncogene, 2009. 28(40): p. 3586-96.

[26] Fachin, AL, SS Mello, P Sandrin-Garcia, et al., Gene expression profiles in human lymphocytes irradiated in vitro with low doses of gamma rays. Radiat Res, 2007. 168(6): p. 650-65.

[27] Tusher, VG, R Tibshirani, and G Chu, Significance analysis of microarrays applied to the ionizing radiation response. Proc Natl Acad Sci U S A, 2001. 98(9): p. 5116-21.

[28] Al-Shahrour, F, P Minguez, JM Vaquerizas, et al., BABELOMICS: a suite of web tools for functional annotation and analysis of groups of genes in high-throughput experiments. Nucleic Acids Res, 2005. 33(Web Server issue): p. W460-4.

[29] Bock, KW and C Kohle, Ah receptor: dioxin-mediated toxic responses as hints to deregulated physiologic functions. Biochem Pharmacol, 2006. 72(4): p. 393-404.

[30] Hayhurst, GP, H Strick-Marchand, C Mulet, et al., Morphogenetic competence of HNF4 alpha-deficient mouse hepatic cells. J Hepatol, 2008. 49(3): p. 384-95.

[31] Huang, TH, T Oka, T Asai, et al., Repression by a differentiation-specific factor of the human cytomegalovirus enhancer. Nucleic Acids Res, 1996. 24(9): p. 1695-701.

[32] Wilsker, D, A Patsialou, PB Dallas, et al., ARID proteins: a diverse family of DNA binding proteins implicated in the control of cell growth, differentiation, and development. Cell Growth Differ, 2002. 13(3): p. 95-106.

[33] Healy, J, C Richer, M Bourgey, et al., Replication analysis confirms the association of ARID5B with childhood B-cell acute lymphoblastic leukemia. Haematologica, 2010. 95(9): p. 1608-11.

[34] Tchougounova, E, Y Jiang, D Brasater, et al., Sox5 can suppress platelet-derived growth factor B-induced glioma development in Ink4a-deficient mice through induction of acute cellular senescence. Oncogene, 2009. 28(12): p. 1537-48.

[35] Honda, N, K Yagi, GR Ding, et al., Radiosensitization by overexpression of the non-phosphorylation form of IkappaB-alpha in human glioma cells. J Radiat Res, 2002. 43(3): p. 283-92.

[36] Yamagishi, N, J Miyakoshi, and H Takebe, Enhanced radiosensitivity by inhibition of nuclear factor kappa B activation in human malignant glioma cells. Int J Radiat Biol, 1997. 72(2): p. 157-62.

[37] Van Esch, H, P Groenen, MA Nesbit, et al., GATA3 haplo-insufficiency causes human HDR syndrome. Nature, 2000. 406(6794): p. 419-22.

[38] Muroya, K, T Hasegawa, Y Ito, et al., GATA3 abnormalities and the phenotypic spectrum of HDR syndrome. J Med Genet, 2001. 38(6): p. 374-80.

[39] van der Vliet, HJ and EE Nieuwenhuis, IPEX as a result of mutations in FOXP3. Clin Dev Immunol, 2007. 2007: p. 89017.

[40] Matsuura, K, Y Yamaguchi, A Osaki, et al., FOXP3 expression of micrometastasis-positive sentinel nodes in breast cancer patients. Oncol Rep, 2009. 22(5): p. 1181-7.

[41] Wolf, D, AM Wolf, H Rumpold, et al., The expression of the regulatory T cell-specific forkhead box transcription factor FoxP3 is associated with poor prognosis in ovarian cancer. Clin Cancer Res, 2005. 11(23): p. 8326-31.

[42] Klemke, CD, B Fritzsching, B Franz, et al., Paucity of FOXP3+ cells in skin and peripheral blood distinguishes Sézary syndrome from other cutaneous T-cell lymphomas. Leukemia, 2006. 20(6): p. 1123-9.

[43] Yuan, XL, L Chen, MX Li, et al., Elevated expression of Foxp3 in tumor-infiltrating Treg cells suppresses T-cell proliferation and contributes to gastric cancer progression in a COX-2-dependent manner. Clin Immunol, 2010. 134(3): p. 277-88.

[44] Wang, L, R Liu, W Li, et al., Somatic single hits inactivate the X-linked tumor suppressor FOXP3 in the prostate. Cancer Cell, 2009. 16(4): p. 336-46.

[45] Steer, HJ, RA Lake, AK Nowak, et al., Harnessing the immune response to treat cancer. Oncogene, 2010. 29(48): p. 6301-13.

[46] Hanash, S, Harnessing the immune response for cancer detection. Cancer Epidemiol Biomarkers Prev, 2011. 20(4): p. 569-70.

[47] Jung, DJ, DH Jin, SW Hong, et al., Foxp3 expression in p53-dependent DNA damage responses. J Biol Chem, 2010. 285(11): p. 7995-8002.

[48] Pérez-Sánchez, C, C Arias-de-la-Fuente, MA Gómez-Ferrería, et al., FHX.L and FHX.S, two isoforms of the human fork-head factor FHX (FOXJ2) with differential activity. J Mol Biol, 2000. 301(4): p. 795-806.

[49] Wang, L, P Wang, Y Liu, et al., Regulation of cellular growth, apoptosis, and Akt activity in human U251 glioma cells by a combination of cisplatin with CRM197. Anticancer Drugs, 2012. 23(1): p. 81-9.

[50] Chen, X, X Cao, G Tao, et al., FOXJ2 expression in rat spinal cord after injury and its role in inflammation. J Mol Neurosci, 2012. 47(1): p. 158-65.

[51] Wang, H, P Iakova, M Wilde, et al., C/EBPalpha arrests cell proliferation through direct inhibition of Cdk2 and Cdk4. Mol Cell, 2001. 8(4): p. 817-28.

[52] Yoon, K and RC Smart, C/EBPalpha is a DNA damage-inducible p53-regulated mediator of the G1 checkpoint in keratinocytes. Mol Cell Biol, 2004. 24(24): p. 10650-60.

[53] Ghosh, AP, BJ Klocke, ME Ballestas, et al., CHOP Potentially Co-Operates with FOXO3a in Neuronal Cells to Regulate PUMA and BIM Expression in Response to ER Stress. PLoS ONE, 2012. 7(6): p. e39586.

[54] Homma, J, R Yamanaka, N Yajima, et al., Increased expression of CCAAT/enhancer binding protein beta correlates with prognosis in glioma patients. Oncol Rep, 2006. 15(3): p. 595-601.

[55] Dahlman, I, M Nilsson, H Jiao, et al., Liver X receptor gene polymorphisms and adipose tissue expression levels in obesity. Pharmacogenet Genomics, 2006. 16(12): p. 881-9.

[56] Chen, Y, Y Tang, S Chen, et al., Regulation of drug resistance by human pregnane X receptor in breast cancer. Cancer Biol Ther, 2009. 8(13): p. 1265-72.

[57] Dotzlaw, H, E Leygue, P Watson, et al., The human orphan receptor PXR messenger RNA is expressed in both normal and neoplastic breast tissue. Clin Cancer Res, 1999. 5(8): p. 2103-7.

[58] Urquhart, BL, RG Tirona, and RB Kim, Nuclear receptors and the regulation of drug-metabolizing enzymes and drug transporters: implications for interindividual variability in response to drugs. J Clin Pharmacol, 2007. 47(5): p. 566-78.

[59] Ding, Y, Y Harada, J Imagawa, et al., AML1/RUNX1 point mutation possibly promotes leukemic transformation in myeloproliferative neoplasms. Blood, 2009. 114(25): p. 5201-5.

[60] Yanagida, M, M Osato, N Yamashita, et al., Increased dosage of Runx1/AML1 acts as a positive modulator of myeloid leukemogenesis in BXH2 mice. Oncogene, 2005. 24(28): p. 4477-85.

[61] Asou, N, The role of a Runt domain transcription factor AML1/RUNX1 in leukemogenesis and its clinical implications. Crit Rev Oncol Hematol, 2003. 45(2): p. 129-50.

[62] Hart, SM and L Foroni, Core binding factor genes and human leukemia. Haematologica, 2002. 87(12): p. 1307-23.

[63] Wang, Q, T Stacy, M Binder, et al., Disruption of the Cbfa2 gene causes necrosis and hemorrhaging in the central nervous system and blocks definitive hematopoiesis. Proc Natl Acad Sci U S A, 1996. 93(8): p. 3444-9.

[64] Satoh, Y, I Matsumura, H Tanaka, et al., C-terminal mutation of RUNX1 attenuates the DNA-damage repair response in hematopoietic stem cells. Leukemia, 2012. 26(2): p. 303-11.

[65]   Umeyama, K, M Watanabe, H Saito, et al., Dominant-negative mutant hepatocyte nuclear factor 1alpha induces diabetes in transgenic-cloned pigs. Transgenic Res, 2009. 18(5): p. 697-706.

[66]   Pal, A, AJ Farmer, C Dudley, et al., Evaluation of serum 1,5 anhydroglucitol levels as a clinical test to differentiate subtypes of diabetes. Diabetes Care, 2010. 33(2): p. 252-7.

[67]   Pinés Corrales, PJ, MP López Garrido, S Aznar Rodríguez, et al., Clinical differences between patients with MODY-3, MODY-2 and type 2 diabetes mellitus with I27L polymorphism in the HNF1alpha gene. Endocrinol Nutr, 2010. 57(1): p. 4-8.

[68]   Rebouissou, S, C Rosty, F Lecuru, et al., Mutation of TCF1 encoding hepatocyte nuclear factor 1alpha in gynecological cancer. Oncogene, 2004. 23(45): p. 7588-92.

[69]   Bélanger, AS, J Tojcic, M Harvey, et al., Regulation of UGT1A1 and HNF1 transcription factor gene expression by DNA methylation in colon cancer cells. BMC Mol Biol, 2010. 11: p. 9.

[70]   Piessen, G, N Jonckheere, A Vincent, et al., Regulation of the human mucin MUC4 by taurodeoxycholic and taurochenodeoxycholic bile acids in oesophageal cancer cells is mediated by hepatocyte nuclear factor 1alpha. Biochem J, 2007. 402(1): p. 81-91.

[71]   Thierry-Mieg, D and J Thierry-Mieg, AceView: a comprehensive cDNA-supported gene and transcripts annotation. Genome Biol, 2006. 7 Suppl 1: p. S12.1-14.

[72]   Najdi, R, A Syed, L Arce, et al., A Wnt kinase network alters nuclear localization of TCF-1 in colon cancer. Oncogene, 2009. 28(47): p. 4133-46.

[73]   Roth, W, C Wild-Bode, M Platten, et al., Secreted Frizzled-related proteins inhibit motility and promote growth of human malignant glioma cells. Oncogene, 2000. 19(37): p. 4210-20.

[74]   DeAlmeida, VI, L Miao, JA Ernst, et al., The soluble wnt receptor Frizzled8CRD-hFc inhibits the growth of teratocarcinomas in vivo. Cancer Res, 2007. 67(11): p. 5371-9.

[75]   deGraffenried, LA, TA Hopp, AJ Valente, et al., Regulation of the estrogen receptor alpha minimal promoter by Sp1, USF-1 and ERalpha. Breast Cancer Res Treat, 2004. 85(2): p. 111-20.

[76]   Baron, Y, S Corre, N Mouchet, et al., USF-1 is critical for maintaining genome integrity in response to UV-induced DNA photolesions. PLoS Genet, 2012. 8(1): p. e1002470.

[77]   Vaninetti, N, L Williams, L Geldenhuys, et al., Regulation of CDX2 expression in esophageal adenocarcinoma. Mol Carcinog, 2009. 48(10): p. 965-74.

[78]   Lord, RV, J Brabender, K Wickramasinghe, et al., Increased CDX2 and decreased PITX1 homeobox gene expression in Barrett's esophagus and Barrett's-associated adenocarcinoma. Surgery, 2005. 138(5): p. 924-31.

[79] Wu, XS, Y Akiyama, T Igari, et al., Expression of homeodomain protein CDX2 in gall-
       bladder carcinomas. J Cancer Res Clin Oncol, 2005. 131(5): p. 271-8.

[80] Ishikawa, A, M Sasaki, S Ohira, et al., Aberrant expression of CDX2 is closely related
       to the intestinal metaplasia and MUC2 expression in intraductal papillary neoplasm
       of the liver in hepatolithiasis. Lab Invest, 2004. 84(5): p. 629-38.

[81] Wong, NA, MP Britton, GS Choi, et al., Loss of CDX1 expression in colorectal carci-
       noma: promoter methylation, mutation, and loss of heterozygosity analyses of 37 cell
       lines. Proc Natl Acad Sci U S A, 2004. 101(2): p. 574-9.

[82] Suh, ER, CS Ha, EB Rankin, et al., DNA methylation down-regulates CDX1 gene ex-
       pression in colorectal cancer cell lines. J Biol Chem, 2002. 277(39): p. 35795-800.

[83] Mallo, GV, H Rechreche, JM Frigerio, et al., Molecular cloning, sequencing and ex-
       pression of the mRNA encoding human Cdx1 and Cdx2 homeobox. Down-regula-
       tion of Cdx1 and Cdx2 mRNA expression during colorectal carcinogenesis. Int J
       Cancer, 1997. 74(1): p. 35-44.

[84] Yeh, TS, YP Ho, CT Chiu, et al., Aberrant expression of cdx2 homeobox gene in intra-
       ductal papillary-mucinous neoplasm of the pancreas but not in pancreatic ductal ad-
       enocarcinoma. Pancreas, 2005. 30(3): p. 233-8.

[85] Ekstrand, AJ and L Zech, Human c-fos proto-oncogene mapped to chromosome 14,
       band q24.3-q31. Possibilities for oncogene activation by chromosomal rearrange-
       ments in human neoplasms. Exp Cell Res, 1987. 169(1): p. 262-6.

[86] Verma, IM, J Deschamps, C Van Beveren, et al., Human fos gene. Cold Spring Harb
       Symp Quant Biol, 1986. 51 Pt 2: p. 949-58.

[87] Kalogeropoulou, M, A Voulgari, V Kostourou, et al., TAF4b and Jun/activating pro-
       tein-1 collaborate to regulate the expression of integrin alpha6 and cancer cell migra-
       tion properties. Mol Cancer Res, 2010. 8(4): p. 554-68.

[88] Sato, N, MD Sadar, N Bruchovsky, et al., Androgenic induction of prostate-specific
       antigen gene is repressed by protein-protein interaction between the androgen recep-
       tor and AP-1/c-Jun in the human prostate cancer cell line LNCaP. J Biol Chem, 1997.
       272(28): p. 17485-94.

[89] Wang, L, Y Sun, M Jiang, et al., FOS proliferating network construction in early col-
       orectal cancer (CRC) based on integrative significant function cluster and inferring
       analysis. Cancer Invest, 2009. 27(8): p. 816-24.

[90] Liu, G, W Ding, X Liu, et al., c-Fos is required for TGFbeta1 production and the asso-
       ciated paracrine migratory effects of human colon carcinoma cells. Mol Carcinog,
       2006. 45(8): p. 582-93.

[91] Konsman, JP and A Blomqvist, Forebrain patterns of c-Fos and FosB induction during cancer-associated anorexia-cachexia in rat. Eur J Neurosci, 2005. 21(10): p. 2752-66.

[92] Endo, M, K Yasui, T Nakajima, et al., Infrequent amplification of JUN in hepatocellular carcinoma. Anticancer Res, 2009. 29(12): p. 4989-94.

[93] Myllykangas, S, O Monni, B Nagy, et al., Helicobacter pylori infection activates FOS and stress-response genes and alters expression of genes in gastric cancer-specific loci. Genes Chromosomes Cancer, 2004. 40(4): p. 334-41.

[94] Dahlman-Wright, K, Y Qiao, P Jonsson, et al., Interplay between AP-1 and estrogen receptor α in regulating gene expression and proliferation networks in breast cancer cells. Carcinogenesis, 2012.

[95] Hamdi, M, HE Popeijus, F Carlotti, et al., ATF3 and Fra1 have opposite functions in JNK- and ERK-dependent DNA damage responses. DNA Repair (Amst), 2008.

[96] Meise, R, MT Tomicic, B Kaina, et al., The chloroethylating anticancer drug ACNU induces FRA1 that is involved in drug resistance of glioma cells. Biochim Biophys Acta, 2012. 1823(7): p. 1199-207.

[97] Choi, D, SM Sharma, S Pasadhika, et al., Application of Biostatistics and Bioinformatics Tools to Identify Putative Transcription Factor-Gene Regulatory Network of Ankylosing Spondylitis and Sarcoidosis. Commun Stat Theory Methods, 2009. 38(18): p. 3326-3338.

[98] Eisen, MB, PT Spellman, PO Brown, et al., Cluster analysis and display of genome wide expression patterns. Proc Natl Acad Sci U S A, 1998. 95(25): p. 14863-8.

[99] Lee, HK, AK Hsu, J Sajdak, et al., Coexpression analysis of human genes across many microarray data sets. Genome Res, 2004. 14(6): p. 1085-94.

[100] Stuart, JM, E Segal, D Koller, et al., A gene-coexpression network for global discovery of conserved genetic modules. Science, 2003. 302(5643): p. 249-55.

[101] Mees, C, J Nemunaitis, and N Senzer, Transcription factors: their potential as targets for an individualized therapeutic approach to cancer. Cancer Gene Ther, 2009. 16(2): p. 103-12.

[102] Huang da, W, BT Sherman, and RA Lempicki, Systematic and integrative analysis of large gene lists using DAVID bioinformatics resources. Nat Protoc, 2009. 4(1): p. 44-57.

[103] Brabec, V and J Kasparkova, Modifications of DNA by platinum complexes. Relation to resistance of tumors to platinum antitumor drugs. Drug Resist Updat, 2005. 8(3): p. 131-46.

[104] Torigoe, T, H Izumi, H Ishiguchi, et al., Cisplatin resistance and transcription factors. Curr Med Chem Anticancer Agents, 2005. 5(1): p. 15-27.

[105] Zhang, P, Z Zhang, X Zhou, et al., Identification of genes associated with cisplatin resistance in human oral squamous cell carcinoma cell line. BMC Cancer, 2006. 6: p. 224.

[106] Jaber, N, Z Dou, JS Chen, et al., Class III PI3K Vps34 plays an essential role in autophagy and in heart and liver function. Proc Natl Acad Sci U S A, 2012. 109(6): p. 2003-8.

[107] Attree, O, IM Olivos, I Okabe, et al., The Lowe's oculocerebrorenal syndrome gene encodes a protein highly homologous to inositol polyphosphate-5-phosphatase. Nature, 1992. 358(6383): p. 239-42.

[108] Damia, G, L Filiberti, F Vikhanskaya, et al., Cisplatinum and taxol induce different patterns of p53 phosphorylation. Neoplasia, 2001. 3(1): p. 10-6.

[109] Yazlovitskaya, EM and DL Persons, Inhibition of cisplatin-induced ATR activity and enhanced sensitivity to cisplatin. Anticancer Res, 2003. 23(3B): p. 2275-9.

[110] Pabla, N, S Huang, QS Mi, et al., ATR-Chk2 signaling in p53 activation and DNA damage response during cisplatin-induced apoptosis. J Biol Chem, 2008. 283(10): p. 6572-83.

[111] Reimer, CL, AM Borras, SK Kurdistani, et al., Altered regulation of cyclin G in human breast cancer and its specific localization at replication foci in response to DNA damage in p53+/+ cells. J Biol Chem, 1999. 274(16): p. 11022-9.

[112] Kato, MV, The mechanisms of death of an erythroleukemic cell line by p53: involvement of the microtubule and mitochondria. Leuk Lymphoma, 1999. 33(1-2): p. 181-6.

[113] Velasco-Miguel, S, L Buckbinder, P Jean, et al., PA26, a novel target of the p53 tumor suppressor and member of the GADD family of DNA damage and growth arrest inducible genes. Oncogene, 1999. 18(1): p. 127-37.

[114] Konopka, G and A Bonni, Signaling pathways regulating gliomagenesis. Curr Mol Med, 2003. 3(1): p. 73-84.

[115] Ishii, N, D Maier, A Merlo, et al., Frequent co-alterations of TP53, p16/CDKN2A, p14ARF, PTEN tumor suppressor genes in human glioma cell lines. Brain Pathol, 1999. 9(3): p. 469-79.

[116] Struhl, K, Gene regulation. A paradigm for precision. Science, 2001. 293(5532): p. 1054-5.

[117] Chen, J, RM McKay, and LF Parada, Malignant glioma: lessons from genomics, mouse models, and stem cells. Cell, 2012. 149(1): p. 36-47.

MicroRNAs

Chapter 3

MicroRNAs Regulated Brain Tumor Cell Phenotype and Their Therapeutic Potential

Chunzhi Zhang, Budong Chen, Xiangying Xu,
Baolin Han, Guangshun Wang and Jinhuan Wang

Additional information is available at the end of the chapter

1. Introduction

MicroRNAs (miRNAs)are short 18–25 nucleotide small non-coding RNA molecules that function to silence gene expression via sophisticated post-transcriptional regulation[1]. Since their discovery in the early 1990s, these small molecules have been shown to play an important regulatory role in a wide range of biological and pathological processes. Over 30% of human messenger RNAs (mRNAs) are regulated by miRNAs[2]. miRNAs generated by the canonical biogenesis pathway are transcribed as precursor RNAs from intergenic, intronic or polycis-tronic genomic loci by RNA polymerase II (Pol II). The primary miRNA (pri-miRNA) transcript forms a stem–loop structure that is recognized and processed by the Drosha and DGCR8 RNase III complex or the spliceosome apparatus in the nucleus. In the non-canonical miRNA pathway, miRNAs are transcribed directly as endogenous short hairpin RNAs (endo-shRNAs) or derive directly through splicing from introns that can refold into hairpins (mirtrons). The trimmed precursor (pre-miRNA) hairpins from both canonical and non-canonical miRNA pathways are then transported by an exportin 5 and RAN-GTP-dependent process to the cytosol, where they are typically further processed by the Dicer and transactivation-response RNA-binding protein (TRBP) RNase III enzyme complex to form the mature double-stranded ~22-nucleotide miRNA. Argonaute proteins (for example, AGO2)

then unwind the miRNA duplex and facilitate incorporation of the miRNA-targeting strand (also known as the guide strand) into the AGO-containing RNA-induced silencing complex (RISC). The RISC– miRNA assembly is then guided to specific target sequences in mRNAs. The initial recognition of mRNAs by the RISC–miRNA complex is driven primarily by Watson–Crick base-pairing of nucleotides 2 to 8 in the mature miRNA (termed the seed sequence) with specific mRNA target sequences chiefly located in the 3' untranslated region, and additional base-pairing affords greater affinity and targeting efficiency(Figure1)[3].

Given the pivotal regulatory role of miRNAs in a broad range of biological processes, it is not surprising that miRNAs play a role in human cancers, including brain tumor. First, about 50% of human miRNAs are located in cancer-associated genomic regions and fragile sites, suggesting that they might be the target genes underlying such aberrant intervals [5]. Second, the advent of high-throughput detection method has promoted expression profiling of miRNAs in normal and tumor tissues. Compared to normal tissues, anomalous levels of miRNA subsets have been found in almost all tumor types examined [6, 7]. Third, miRNAs with tumor-suppressive gene and oncogene-like properties have been described.

Since the first description of aberrant miRNA expression in glioblastomas and pituitary adenomas in 2005 [8, 9], there have been increasing reports each year about miRNA deregulation and function in various brain tumors. In this chapter, we summarize the current findings of miRNA study in brain cancers and discuss the diagnostic and therapeutic potential of miRNAs, mainly in glioma.

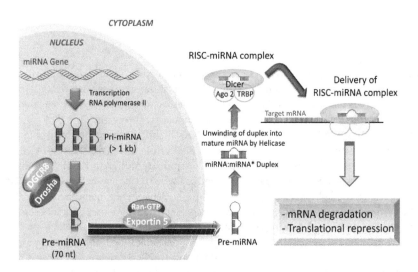

Figure 1. The miRNA biogenesis pathway[4]

2. MiRNAs profile in brain tumor

CBTRUS obtained incidence data from 48 population-based cancer registries that include cases of malignant and non–malignant (benign and uncertain) primary brain and central nervous system tumors in the United States in 2004-2007. The most frequently reported histology is the predominately non–malignant meningioma, which accounts for 34% of all tumors, followed by glioblastoma (17%). The predominately non-malignant pituitary and nerve sheath tumors account for 13% and 9% of all tumors, respectively. Acoustic neuromas (defined by ICD-O-3 site code C72.4 and histology code 9560) account for 63% of all nerve sheath tumors(Figure2).

Only recently, the miRNAs attracted increasing attention as potential diagnostic or even therapeutic tools in brain tumors. Profiling techniques to identify global expression patterns of miRNAs in brain tumors have been widely used to uncover aberrantly expressed micro-RNAs in tumor genomes. Ciafrè et al. found nine (miR-10b, miR-130a, miR-221, miR-125b-1, miR-125b-2, miR-9-2, miR-21, miR-25, miR-123) and four miRNAs (miR-128a, miR-181c, miR-181a, miR-181b), respectively, out of 245 miRNAs to be up-/down-regulated in human glioblastoma samples, and nine (miR-221, miR-23a, miR-24-2, miR-24-1, miR-23b, miR-21,miR-222-prec, miR-191, miR-220) and seven miRNAs(miR-181a, miR-181b, miR-128b, miR-197, miR-181c,miR-125b-2, miR-125b-1), respectively, to be up-/down-regulated in human glioblastoma cell lines[10]. Chan et al.[8] demonstrated five (miR-21, miR-138, miR-347, miR-291-5', miR-135) and three miRNAs (miR-198, miR-188,miR-202), respectively, out of 180 miRNAs to be up- and downregulated in glioblastoma samples. Sasayama et al.[11] found miR-10b, miR-21, miR-183, miR-92b and miR-106b to be up-, and miR- 302c*, miR-379, miR-329, miR-134 and miR-369-3p to be downregulated in human glioblastoma samples. Other studies reported several miRNAs to be significantly deregulated in glioma samples of Chinese patients (including miR-34a, miR-15b, miR-200a and miR-146b) [12], or miR-29b, miR-125a and miR-149 to be downregulated in glioblastomas [13]. In an array study with 192 miRNAs, 13 miRNAs (miR-101, miR-128a, miR-132, miR-133a, miR-133b, miR-149, miR-153, miR-154*, miR-185, miR-29b, miR-323, miR-328, miR-330) were found to be downregulated and three miRNAs to be upregulated (miR-21, miR-155, miR-210) in glioblastoma multiforme [14]. Another micro-array study identified 55 miRNAs out of 756 miRNAs to be upregulated and 29miRNAs to be downregulated in malignant astrocytomas (primary and secondary glioblastoma and ana-plastic astrocytoma, respectively) compared to controls [15].

In additional to gliomas, miRNA profiling also had been discovered in some other brain tumors. Ferretti et al were the first to identify signatures of a set of 248 miRNAs in a panel of primary medulloblastomas and normal cerebellar controls using high throughput expression profiles. They showed different expression profiles between normal brain and tumor and between distinct tumor histotypes. In particular, they detected an upregulation of mir-21 and miR-17-92 cluster (miR-17-5p, miR-20a and miR-19a) and a downregulation of miR-128a/b, let-7, miR-124a, miR-103, miR-134, miR-138, miR-149, miR-181b, miR-9 and miR-125a, most of them previously reported to be dysregulated in other brain tumor cell lines or nervous system cancers [16]. Moreover, Recent microarray data reported a possible role of miRNAs in pituitary adenomas. The first connection between pituitary adenomas and miRNAs was established by Bottoni et al in 2005, that showed a downregulation of mir-15a and miR-16-1 in GH-secreting and in PRL-secreting adenomas compared to normal pituitary tissue[8]. In 2007 Bottoni et al explored the miRNAome of pituitary tumors by microarray. They found that 30 miRNAs are differentially expressed between normal pituitary gland and pituitary adenomas. Among them, miR-150, miR-152, miR-191, and miR-192 were found to be upregulated in pituitary

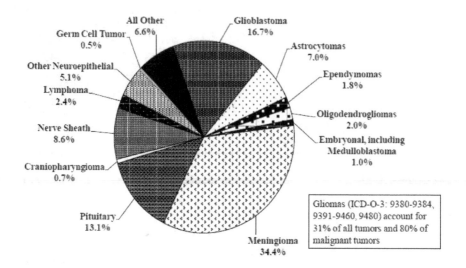

Figure 2. Distribution of All Primary Brain and CNS Tumors by Histology (N=226,791) CBTRUS Statistical Report: NPCR and SEER Data from 2004-2007

adenomas, and miR-132, miR-128a, miR-136, miR-16-1, and let-7 are downregulated[17]. As for meningioma, Feng Zhi et al found a list of 14 miRNAs that were differentially expressed in meningioma compared to normal adjacent tissue(NAT)samples. Twelve miRNAs, including miR-17-5p, miR-22-3p, miR-24-3p, miR-26b-5p, miR-27a-3p, miR-27b-3p, miR-96-5p, miR-146a-5p, miR-155-5p, miR-186-5p, miR-190a and miR-199a were shown to be upregulated by a factor greater than twofold, whereas two miRNAs, including miR-29c-3p and miR-219-5p, were significantly downregulated[18].

3. Abberant miRNAs as prognostic and/or diagnostic marker for brain tumor patients

The use of miRNAs as tumor biomarkers has gained growing interest in the last few years. Accumulating evidence indicates that miRNA expression can be used as a prognostic and/or diagnostic marker for brain tumor patients. Niyazi et al. separated 35 glioblastoma patients into long- and short-term survivors. Then, they found that some miRNAs were significantly different in two group, including miR-3163, miR-539, miR-1305, miR-1260 and let-7a. this is the first dataset defining a prognostic role of miRNA expression patterns in patients with glioblastoma[19]. Moreover, Ma also identified that MiR-196b is overexpressed and confers a poor prognosis via promoting cellular proliferation in glioblastoma patients[20]. Costa et al identified miRNAs that are over-expressed in ependymomas, such as miR-135a and miR-17-5p, and downregulated, such as miR-383 and miR-485-5p. We have also uncovered associations between expression of specific miRNAs which portend a worse prognosis. For example, we have identified a cluster of miRNAs on human chromosome 14q32 that is associated with time to relapse. We also found that miR-203 is an independent marker for relapse compared to the parameters that are currently used. Additionally, we have identified three miRNAs (let-7d, miR-596 and miR-367) that strongly correlate to overall survival[21].

4. Deregulated miRNAs regulated brain tumor cell phenotype

Increasing evidence supports the supposition that miRNAs play an important role in different types of cancers and in various aspects of cancer biology. Abnormal miR levels in tumors have important pathogenetic consequences: miRNAs may act as oncogenes or suppressor genes[22]. For examples, Calin et al. [23] identified two clustered miRNAs (miR-15a and miR-16-1) on the minimal deletion region of chromosome 13q14 and showed that the levels of these miRNAs were significantly reduced in the majority (68%) of B-cell chronic lymphocytic leukemia (CLL). Both miRNAs target the anti-apoptotic gene BCL2, which is frequently overexpressed in CLL [24]. These findings indicate that downregulation of miR-15a and miR-16-1 elevates BCL2 level, contributing to CLL formation and suggesting a tumor-suppressive role for both miRNAs. In contrast, miR-17-92 showed marked upregulation in B-cell lymphomas. Enforced expression of miR-17-92 cluster acted with c-myc to accelerate the onset of B-cell lymphoma in a mouse model [25]. The data suggest that miR-17-92 cluster is a potential oncogene.

Recent evidence supports the ability of miRNAs to regulate brain tumor cell phenotype. We had done some work to identified that miR-221 and miR-222 regulated their target expression to co-modulated glioma cell phenotype, including proliferation, cell cycle, apoptosis and invasion(Figure3)[26-28], and so on.

MiRNAs also regulated radio- and chemo-resistence of glioma. Hierarchical clustering analysis of expression 1100 miRNAs in three glioma cell lines treated with clinically relevant doses of radiation (2Gy) revealed significant (3-4 fold) up-regulation of several miRNA that are implicated in stimulation of survival and proliferation of tumor cells [29]. The set of up-regulated miRNAs includes miR-1285, miR-151-5p, and miR-24-1 that display beneficial effects on tumors by inhibiting the core tumor suppressor p53 (miR-1285) and supporting migration, local metastasis (miR-151-5p), and antiapoptosis (miR-24-1) [30]. Overall, activation of these miRNAs might possibly increase tumor radioresistance in subsequent radiotherapy sessions and stimulate motility of cancer cells thereby at least partially explaining the evidence on enhanced migration of malignant glioma cells in response to radiotherapy [31]. The radiation treatment of glioma cell lines with normal capacity to repair radiation-induced double strand breaks (DSB) of DNA caused activation of let-7 [29], a family of miRNA that suppresses proliferation of gliomblastoma cells [30] (Fig. 4). In contrast, in the radiosensitive human glioma cell line M059J that is deficient in DNA-dependent protein kinase (DNA-PK) and has a low activity of ATM, two key members of the non-homologous end joining pathway of DNA-DSB repair, let-7 miRNA was down-regulated [30].

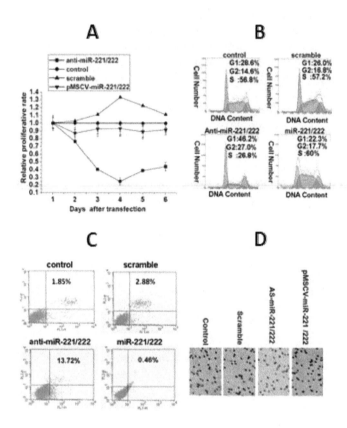

Figure 3. miR-221 and miR-222 regulated their target expression to co-modulated glioma cell phenotype. (A: MTT assay show that knockdown of miR-221/222 lowed proliferated rate of glioma cell; B: knockdown of miR-221/222 induce G1 arrest in glioma cell ;C: Annexin V analysis showed that knockdown of miR-221/222 significantly increased glioma cell apoptosis; D: The transwell assay revealed that knockdown of miR-221/222 significantly decreased glioma cell invasion.

Moreover, MiRNAs were shown to be also involved in the regulation of chemoresistence of glioma by modulating some relevant proteins that are involved in drug metabolism and drug transporter. MiRNAs also affect chemotherapeutic agents induced DNA damage repair (Fig. 4).

5. MiRNAs in gliomas and glioblastoma

MiRNAs affect biological character of varies cells by regulating their targets. So, deregulated miRNAs regulated brain tumor cell phenotype by regulating their targets, including proliferation, cell cycle, apoptosis, invasion, and so on.

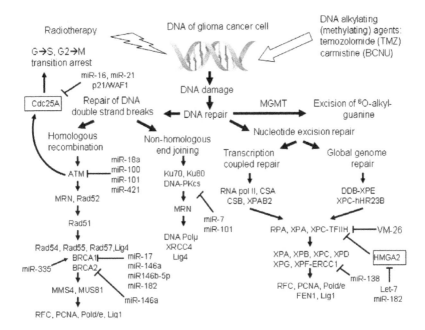

Figure 4. MicroRNAs are involved in the regulation of DNA repair in cancer cells after treatment with ionizing radiation (radiotherapy) and DNA alkylating drugs such as temozolomide and carmistine[30].

5.1. MiR-221 and miR-222

MiR-221 and miR-222 are both up-regulated in several glioma derived cell lines and in glioma samples [26-28]. They are clustered within a 1-kb genomic interval on chromosome X, so they could be generated from the same primary transcript [26].

Two members of the Kip/Cip family of CDK inhibitors and key negative regulators of the cell cycle, p57 and p27, have been identified as putative direct targets of these miRNAs. According to this theory, the 3'-UTR of p57 harbors one site expected to be recognized by both miR-221 and miR-222, whereas the 3'-UTR of p27 contains two sites for both miRNAs. Transfection of both miR-221 and miR-222 greatly reduce the levels of p57 and p27 proteins, while downregulation of either microRNA 221 or 222 in glioblastoma cells caused an increase in p27 levels and enhanced expression of the luciferase reporter gene fused to the p27 3'-UTR. These results suggest that miR-221 and miR-222 could promote cell proliferation and S-phase entry together with further cooperative events and that miRNA 221 and 222 inhibition may be a potential therapeutic target to reduce the aggressive growth of glioblastoma by restoring normal levels of their target proteins [32]. The inverse correlation between mir-221/222 and p27 levels, the impairment of growth potential and the G1 to S shift in the cell cycle of glioma cells after inhibition of mir-221/222, were later confirmed by Zhang et al. They extended their study to in vivo trials and showed that miR-221/222 knocked-down through antisense oligonucleotides strongly reduced glioma subcutaneous mice xenografts growth through up regulation of p27 [26] and enhanced radiosensitivity of glioblastoma cell lines [33]. Further evidence showed that knockdown of miR-221/222 induced a change of mitochondrial membrane potential and caspase-mediated apoptosis on glioblastoma cells. Indeed, mir-221/222 directly downregulate the proapoptotic protein PUMA, which leads in turn to decrease Bcl-2 and increase BAX. these results confirm the oncogenic role of mir-221/222 on glioblastoma [27]. Our recent studies identified that mir-221/222 increased cell invasion and reduced gap junction intercellular communication (GJIC) by regulating TIMP3 and Cx43[28,34].

5.2. MiR-21

Microarray profiling studies, further validated by Northern blotting qRT-PCR and real-time PCR analysis, showed that miRNA-21 is strongly elevated in glioma and glioblastoma tumor samples and glioma cell lines when compared to non-neoplastic control samples, and upregulation is particularly prominent in grade IV astrocytomas [35-37]. High expression of miR-21 was significantly associated with poor patient survival, suggesting that, in combination with other aberrant expressed miRNAs (low expression of miR-181b or miR-106a), miRNA-21 profiling has potential application as novel diagnostic and prognostic indicator [37].

Suppression of mir-21 in glioblastoma cells decreased the metabolic activity of cell culture and cell number, and was associated with a marked increase in apoptosis and caspase activation [35]. MiR-21 knockdown also leads to a considerable reduction of glioma volumes in mouse xenografts [38]. Knockdown mir-21 inhibited proliferation and cell invasion and induced apoptosis through the activation of caspase-3 and -9 in glioma cell lines, which may be related to a mir-21-dependent modulation of multiple potential target genes, such as TIMP3 [39,40].

From an in silico constructed study of miR-21 predicted targets and further pathway analysis of computer generated lists of the identified target genes, emerged that mir-21 targets multiple components of the p53, transforming growth factor-β (TGF-β) and mitochondrial apoptosis pathways, that contribute to its tumor promoting and antiapoptotic activity. The phenotypic effects observed upon downregulation of miR-21 in glioblastoma cells, reflect the repression of these pathways and result in significant increase in apoptotic cells, reduced growth and cell cycle arrest at G0-G1 [41]. Further bioinformatics analysis evidenced that multiple genes involved in apoptosis pathways (such as PDCD4, MTAP, and SOX5), carry putative miR-21 binding sites. PDCD4 mRNA is a direct functional target of miR-21 and its expression inversely correlates with mir-21 in a number of glioblastoma cell lines (T98G, A172, U87, and U251). Consistent with these observations, downregulation of mir-21 restored protein level of PDCD4 while, ectopic overexpression of mir-21, inhibits PDCD4-dependent apoptosis [42]. Mir-21 controls tumor invasiveness and microvascular proliferation by regulating the expression of two of the major inhibitors of matrix metalloproteinases (MMPs): RECK and TIMP3. Mir-21 knockdown decreases RECK and TIMP3 protein levels and MMPs activity both in vivo and in vitro leading to a reduction of glioma cell motility and invasion [43]. Although PTEN tumor suppressor gene has been validated as a miR-21 target by computational analysis, downregulation of mir-21 leads to an inhibition of tumor growth in glioblastoma cell lines and xenograft tumors independently of PTEN mutational status [44,45]. MiRNA expression profile scanning data after inhibition of miR-21, strongly indicated that BID, FAS, PRS6, and SOCS4 tumor suppressor genes were upregulated and evidenced a suppression of EGFR, activated Akt, cyclin D, and Bcl-2. This study highlighted that miR-21 targets multiple pathways responsible of inhibition of glioma growth in absence of PTEN [46].

Further findings strengthened the hypothesis that miR-21 represents a promising target to improve the efficacy of chemotherapy. In a recent study mir-21 was shown to play a key role in promoting human glioblastoma cells U87MG resistance against the antitumoral agent temozolomide (TMZ). Indeed, ectopic overexpression of mir-21 significantly reduced TMZ-induced apoptosis in this cell line through a suppression of Bax/Bcl-2 ratio and caspase-3 activity. These results confirm the hypothesis that mir-21 overexpression during glioma progression could be responsible of clinical resistance to chemotherapy with the promising alkylating agent TMZ [47]. Li et al demonstrated that mir-21 is also involved in glioblastoma cell chemoresistance to the chemotherapeutic agent VM-26, as shown by the observation that miR-21 knockdown sensitized GBM cells to VM-26. This is likely to happen because mir-21 regulates and inhibit LRRFIP1 gene expression by direct interaction [48]. This gene encodes a protein, also known as the TRAF-interacting protein (TRIP), that inhibits NF-κB signaling, a pathway that is known to be responsible for protection against apoptosis [49] and tumor chemoresistance [50]. Additionally, suppression of miRNA-21 expression in glioblastoma cell lines enhances sensitivity of cancer cells to antineoplastic cytotoxic therapy with neural precursor cells (NPC) expressing a secretable variant of the cytotoxic agent tumor necrosis factor related apoptosis inducing ligand (S-TRAIL). The synergistic effect was observed both in vitro, through an increased caspase associated cytotoxic death, and in vivo, where miR-21 knockdown and NPC-mediated S-TRAIL reduce cancer growth in tumor xenografts [38]. A recent study that evaluated the potential role of mir-21 as a therapeutic tool to enhance the cytotoxic effect of standard chemotherapy showed that co-delivery of miR-21 and 5-fluorouracil (5-FU) by using a poly(amidoamine) (PAMAM) dendrimer as a carrier, significantly improved the cytotoxicity of the antitumor agent leading to an higher apoptosis rate and a reduction of the migration ability of tumor cells [51]. Finally, downregulation of miR-21, contributes to the antitumor effects of IFN-β on glioma cell and intracranial tumor xenografts and the activation of the transcription factor STAT3 may have a key role in the IFN-β mediated suppression of mir-21 [52].

5.3. Mir-34a

Mir-34a, transcriptional target of p53 located within chromosome 1p36, has been proposed as a potential tumor suppressor. MiR-34a is also downregulated in glioblastoma tissues and cell lines compared to normal brain tissues and is markedly reduced in p53-mutant cells compared to cells expressing wild-type p53 [53,54].

MiR-34a possesses hundreds of predicted mRNA targets which could mediate its inhibitory effects on tumor growth. A few of these have been experimentally verified and include oncogenes such as MYC, CCND1, CDK6, SIRT1 [55] and c-Met [56]. It was shown to directly inhibit c-Met in glioma and medulloblastoma cells and Notch-1/Notch-2 in glioma cells and stem cells by binding to the 3'-UTRs of their mRNA. Furthermore, mir-34a inversely correlates with c-Met, Notch1, Notch2 and CDK6 protein expression in glioma cells. Transfection of microRNA34a in brain tumor cells strongly inhibits cell proliferation, cell cycle progression, cell survival, cell invasion, and in vivo glioma xenograft growth but do not affect cell cycle or death when transfected to human astrocytes, which showed normal expression levels of microRNA 34a. Restoration of c-Met or Notch-1 and Notch-2 expression by constructs lacking 3'-UTR regions partially reverted cell cycle arrest and apoptosis induced by miR-34a in glioma cells or stem cells, confirming the hypothesis that the antitumor effects of miR-34a are achieved via targeting of multiple oncogenes [53]. Interestingly, mir-34a also affect glioma stem cell differentiation and growth. Luan et al recently reported silent information regulator 1 (Sirt1) as a direct negative target of mir34a in glioma cell lines at a posttranscriptional level [54]. Sirt1 is a NAD-dependent deacetylase that regulates apoptosis in response to oxidative and genotoxic stress, and has recently been involved in tumorigenesis acting as an oncogene [57].

5.4. Mir-128

Mir-128, a brain enriched microRNA, is downregulated in glioma cell lines and tissue when compared to normal brain samples [58]. Mir-128 overexpression decreased glioma cell proliferation in vitro and glioma xenograft growth in vivo, and is inversely correlated to Bmi-1 expression. Mir-128 directly targets and downregulates Bmi-1 by binding its 3'-UTR region [59] and leads to a concomitant overexpression of p21CIP1 and a decrease in phosphorylated Akt [58]. Bmi-1 expression is a critical factor of normal stem cell maintenance and glioblastoma self-renewal and loss of Bmi-1-mediated self-renewal of neural stem cells has been shown to be associated with upregulation of p21CIP1 [60] and decreased Akt activation [61]. Consistently with these observations, miR-128 overexpression in human glioma neurosphere cultures possessing a glioma 'stem-like' cell phenotype, evidenced that miR-128 specifically blocked glioma self-renewal reducing neurosphere number and size. In conclusion, mir-128 downregulation is likely to enhance glioma tumorigenesis by promoting an undifferentiated phenotype and self renewing state through Bmi-1 increased expression [58]. By bioinformatical analysis, E2F3a, a transcription factor involved in cell cycle progression [62], has been identified as a direct target of this miRNA. Indeed, Mir-128 and E2F3a levels are negatively correlated and mir-128 overexpression has similar inhibitory effects on proliferation of glioma cell lines as E2F3a knocking down Ectopic overexpression of E2F3a partially reversed the effects of mir-128, suggesting that mir-128 could exert its antitumor effects at least partially by inhibiting E2F3a expression. Among its target genes angiopoietin-related protein 5 (ARP5) was identified with bioinformatical tools and then confirmed to be inversely correlated to mir-128 levels in glioblastoma cells and tissue and downregulated after ectopic overexpression of this miRNA [58]. ARP5 seems to be a key regulator of cell proliferation, remodeling and regeneration [63] and could be a member of a group of genes regulated by mir-128 that coordinately contribute to glioma and GBM pathology [59].

5.5. Mir-451

Mir-451 was found to be upregulated in glioma samples compared to normal brain on microarray-based miRNAome profiling [64]. MiR-451 showed a striking spatial distribution, with groups of positive cells concentrated around a subset of blood vessels. Moreover, high levels of mir-451 are correlated to a poor prognosis in glioma patients. Mir-451 could regulate the balance of proliferation and migration in glioma cells in response to changes in glucose levels and metabolic stress. It regulates 5'-adenosine monophosphate activated protein kinase (AMPK) pathway in response to glucose levels in glioma cells, through the modulation of the activity of its upstream activator LKB1 [65]. Activation of LKB1 is a potent anti-proliferative signal, and also influences cell polarity, a process known to affect cell motility [66].

MiR-451 regulates LKB1 activity by directly targeting CAB39, a component of the active LKB1complex, leading to a downregulation of CAB39 protein levels. Down-regulation of mir-451 levels in response to glucose deprivation leads to intense activation of LKB1 and downstream pathways, allowing cells to survive metabolic stress and promoting cancer cell migration. Conversely, when glucose is sufficient, elevated miR-451 levels lead to reduced LKB1/AMPK pathway activation. This facilitates cell proliferation but makes cells more sensitive to glucose deprivation. Thus mir-451 could be a key regulator of adaptive response of cancer cells to altered energy availability [65].

In partial contrast with these studies a recent report found mir-451 to be downregulated in glioma cell lines. Transfection of mir-451 to glioma cell lines was able to inhibit cell growth, induced G0/G1 phase arrest, increased cell apoptosis and most notably diminished the invasive capacity of these cells as evidenced by transwell invasion assay. These tumor suppressive effects may be due to modulated expression of a panel of proteins including CyclinD1, p27, MMP 2/9 and Bcl-2, probably via regulation of the PI3K/AKT signaling pathway. Indeed, expression of Akt1 protein decreased after mir-451 transfection [67].

5.6. Mir-7

Mir-7, a miRNA modulated during neural differentiation of embryonic stem cells is a putative tumor suppressor gene in glioblastoma. It inhibits EGFR gene expression by directly binding its mRNA at 3'-UTR. Furthermore, miRNA-7 suppresses the activation of Akt pathway and reduces phospho-Akt levels by directly targeting its upstream regulators IRS-1 and IRS-2 [68]. They also identified Raf1 as a direct target of miR-7 by microarray analysis, Western blot and luciferase reporter assays of glioblastoma cells transfected with miR-7 [69]. Inhibition of Akt activation seems to occur independently of mir-7-mediated repression of EGFR pathway. Consistenly with these findings miRNA-7 was markedly downregulated in glioblastoma tissue when compared to normal brain. The proposed mechanism that explains the lower expression of this miRNA is a processing defect in generating pre-miR-7 from pri-miR-7 in glioblastoma. Pre-miRNA-7 transfection decreased viability and invasiveness of glioblastoma lines and glioblastoma derived stem cells and led to an increase in the sub-G0 apoptotic fraction, a decrease in the S fraction and determined a G2-M arrest, most likely by affecting EGFR and Akt pathways, which have an established key role in gliomagenesis [68]. Indeed, EGFR is frequently amplified and highly expressed in glioblastomas [26]. In a recent report mir-7 was also shown to directly inhibit p21-activated kinase 1 (Pak1) in non-brain cancer cells [70]. Pak1 is a widely upregulated signaling kinase in multiple human cancers, and it is involved in the regulation of many signaling pathways, including EGFR and Akt, thus interfering with cell motility, proliferation, and apoptosis [71]. Furthermore, in glioblastomas, PAK1 upregulation is a negative prognostic marker and its knockdown results in impaired cell invasion [72]. These preliminary results suggest mir-7 could have a potential and promising therapeutic role in brain tumors.

5.7. Mir-181

Mir-181a and mir-181b are well known brain-enriched miRNAs [73]. Downregulation of mir-181a and mir-181b was detected in both glioma samples and cell lines [74]. Transfection of both these miRNAs on glioma cell lines results in cell growth inhibition, invasion reduction and apoptosis induction, miR-181b being more effective than miR-181a [74]. In a recent miRNA expression profiling conducted on a set of 124 astrocytoma samples and 60 normal adjacent tissue samples by qRT-PCR, Zhi et al found that downregulation of miR-181b is significantly associated with poor patient survival independently of other clinicopathological factors. Thus, mir-181b has a great potential for being used as a diagnostic and prognostic marker and to better select patients for adjuvant therapy [39].

In a recent study MiR-181b and miR-181c downregulation was found to be significantly associated to a positive response to concomitant chemoradiotherapy with temozolomide in glioblastoma patients, suggesting they could be used as predictive factors for therapy efficacy [75].

5.8. Mir-124/137

MiRNA-124 and miRNA-137 are downregulated in anaplastic astrocytomas and glioblastoma multiforme relative to non-neoplastic brain tissue [9-10]. Consequently, growth factor signaling could promote brain tumor formation through suppression of miR-124 and/or miR-137 expression and inhibition of neural stem cells/tumor stem cell differentiation. Transfection of mir-124 and mir-137 to neural stem cells and tumor-derived stem cells leads to induction of cellular markers of differentiation, G1 cell cycle arrest and reductions of the expression of the cell cycle regulator CDK6, a direct target of both miRNAs. These changes are accompanied by reduced self-renewal and tumorigenicity. Overexpression of miR-124 or miR-137 also reduced the expression of phosphorylated RB, a downstream target of CDK6 [76]. These results suggest that ectopic expression of miRNA-124 and miRNA-137 could represent a valid therapy for glioblastoma multiforme treatment inducing differentiation of tumor cells and cell cycle arrest.

5.9. MiR-125

Mir-125b downregulated in glioma cell lines after treatment with ATRA (all-trans-retinoic acid), a regulator of neural differentiation and proliferation. Ectopic overexpression of mir-125b stimulated glioma cell proliferation, partially recovering the cell growth inhibition induced by ATRA treatment, while mir-125b knockdown promoted ATRA-mediated cell apoptosis. Furthermore, Bmf was identified as a direct target of miR-125b, and they are inversely correlated [77]. Bmf interacts with the prosurvival Bcl-2 proteins, regulating cellular apoptotic pathways [78]. Indeed, transfection with miR-125b increase BCL-2 levels in glioma cells, and expression of BCL-2 was significantly decreased when cells were transfected with miR-125b inhibitor. Thus, Bmf may play an important role in the process of miR-125b influencing cell apoptosis [77].

Recently, Cortez et al identified that mir-125a downregulated in glioblastomas and particulary in glioma stem cells CD133+. Overexpression of mir-125a inhibits invasion properties of glioblastomas, probably through a direct downregulation of podoplanin (PDPN), a membrane sialo-glycoprotein related to invasion and malignancy [79].

5.10. MiR-326

Kefas et al evidenced a feedback loop between miRNA-326 and Notch pathway, frequently deregulated in gliomas. Notch-1 knockdown induced mir-326 upregulation in glioma stem cells, and ectopic overexpression of mir-326 decreased Notch pathway members level and activity. Forced expression of mir-326 also inhibited cell proliferation, viability and invasiveness and induced apoptosis in both established and stem cell-like glioma lines, these effects are at least partially explained through downregulation of the Notch pathway. Moreover, it reduced tumorigenicity in mouse glioma xenografts. Together with the observation that mir-326 is downregulated in glioblastomas, these findings suggest that miR-326 is a potential tumor suppressor in glioma cells and that reversing Notch/miR-326 axis toward miR-326 prevalence appears to be a potential therapy for brain tumors [80].

5.11. Mir-26a

Mir-26a up-regulated in high-grade gliomas. MiR-26a is a direct negative regulator of PTEN and significantly represses PTEN expression. MiR-26a overexpression was attributed to the amplification of miR-26a-2 locus (chromosome 12q), one of the two miR-26a loci present in the human genome (mir-26a-1 and miR-26a-2) and is correlated with monoallelic PTEN deletion. It was suggested a temporal sequence to the molecular evolution of miR-26a-amplified gliomas, with PTEN loss most likely preceding miR-26a-2 amplification and, concordantly, miR-26a overexpression in genetically engineered PTEN+/- mice precluded loss of their remaining PTEN allele. Amplification of mir-26a is likely to promote the silencing of the remaing PTEN transcript in PTEN+/- tumors, event analogous to a loss of heterozygosity. Furthermore, in a murine glioma model, PTEN repression mediated by overexpression of miR-26a, enhanced de novo tumor formation. Akt pathway activation and suppression of its negative regulator PTEN are particularly important and frequently occur in glioma development. These observations document a new epigenetic mechanism for PTEN regulation in gliomagenesis, further highlighting that dysregulation of Akt signaling is crucial to the glioma development and could be modulated through manipulation of miRNA expression [64]. Moreover, MiR-26a is a frequent target of the 12q13.3-14.1 amplicon that also contain CDK4 and CENTG1, two oncogenes that regulate the RB1 and PI3 kinase/AKT pathways, respectively. The presence of this amplification is negatively correlated to patient survival. PTEN, RB1, and MAP3K2/MEKK2 were detected as functional targets of mir-26a in glioblastoma. Ectopic overexpression of miR-26a increased GBM cell growth, decreased apoptosis and enhanced gliomagenesis in vivo. Thus, miR-26a decreases PTEN expression, activates AKT, and promotes tumor growth. Using human U87 GBM cells that lack functional PTEN, mir-26a overexpression increased cell growth and decreased apoptosis despite the absence of PTEN, most probably by downregulating RB1 and MAP3K2, a gene that encodes MEKK2[81]. MEKK2 is a mitogen-activated protein kinase kinase involved in JNK activation pathway that promote apoptosis in GBM cells [82].

5.12. Mir-10b

Mir-10b is upregulated in glioma samples and glioma cell lines compared to non-neoplastic brain tissues. RhoC and urokinasetype plasminogen activator receptor (uPAR), which are known to contribute to glioma invasion and migration, were correlated with mir-10b expression in gliomas, probably via inhibition of the translation of the mRNA encoding homeobox D10 (HOXD10), which in turn represses the expression of these genes [83]. These results suggest that mir-10 could be involved in regulation of the invasion and migration abilities of gliomas.

5.13. Mir-15b

Mir-15b was shown to be elevated in a panel of glioma cell lines. Transfection of glioma cells with miR-15b significantly increased G0/G1 cells and decreased the percentage of cells in S phase, while inhibition of mir-15b increased G0/G1 cell amount. Thus, miR-15b regulates cell cycle progression in glioma cells by targeting cell cycle-related factors as CCNE1 (cyclin E1], a validated downstream target of mir-15b [84].

5.14. Mir-146b

Mir-146b, a miRNA found to be downregulated in human glioma tissue, could exert an antitumor activity by reducing the expression of a matrix metalloproteinase gene, MMP16, one of its direct downstream targets. Indeed, transfection of U373 glioma cells with miR-146b precursor decreased tumor cell migration and invasion, while inhibition of miR-146b by LNA modified anti-miR-146b produced the opposite effect, without affecting cell proliferation [85].

5.15. Mir-296

Recent studies support a role of mir-296 in promoting angiogenesis in gliomas. When brain microvascular endothelial cells were co-cultured with U87 glioma cells or when vascular endothelial growth factor (VEGF) was added to cultured human brain microvascular endothelial cells, miR-296 was upregulated. Moreover, mir-296 levels were higher in endothelial cells isolated from human brain tumors compared to normal brain endothelial cells. Downregulation of miR-296 in endothelial cells resulted in the inhibition of morphologic characteristics associated with angiogenesis and reduced angiogenesis in glioma xenografts in vivo. This probably happens through the downregulation of the hepatocyte growth factor-regulated tyrosine kinase substrate (HGS), a validated target of mir-296, thus leading to a reduced HGS-mediated degradation of the platelet derived growth factor receptor (PDGFR) and vascular endothelial growth factor receptor (VEGFR). This result points out an interesting feedback loop, where VEGF induces miR-296 expression, which in turn increases cell response to VEGF. Consequently, manipulating mir-296 expression, could enable to control a key step in cancer angiogenesis [86].

5.16. Mir-29

Mir-29b was found to be significantly downregulated in glioblastoma samples and cells and CD133+ tumor stem cells. Forced overexpression of this miRNA inhibited invasion and proliferation and induced apoptosis in glioblastoma cells. Mir-29b as well mir-125a directly targets podoplanin (PDPN), a putative marker of neural stem cells, related to invasion and malignancy in glioblastoma [13].

5.17. MiR-17-92 cluster

MiR-17-92 cluster, located within the locus 13q31-q32, encloses five miRNAs (miR-92-1, miR-19a, miR-20a, miR-19b, miR-17-5p), which have been frequently involved in tumorigenesis [87]. This cluster was detected to be amplified in glioblastoma samples. Furthermore, expression of miR-17-92 cluster is downregulated upon induction of differentiation of GBM spheroid cultures by using ATRA. Induction of differentiation leads to deregulation of most of the key pathways associated with self-renewal such as insulin-like growth factor 1 signaling, vitamin D receptor/retinoic acid X receptor activation, Wnt/β-catenin signaling and retinoic acid receptor activation. Inhibition of miR-17-92 cluster leads to decreased cell viability and decreased cell proliferation probably through a de-repression of CDKN1, E2F1, PTEN and CTGF which are upregulated. Particularly, connective tissue growth factor (CTGF) gene was shown to be a direct target of miR-17-92 in glioblastoma spheroids by luciferase reporter assays [88]. CTGF binds vascular endothelial growth factor (VEGFA), which is a central mediator of angiogenesis [89], and inhibits VEGFA-induced angiogenesis [90]. Conversely, VEGFA was shown to inhibit MiR-17-92 [91], thus explaining the concomitant downregulation of VEGFA and miR-17-92 upon induction of differentiation. In conclusion, the interaction between CTGF, VEGFA and miR-17-92 might have a key role in gliomagenesis by targeting multiple regulatory pathways [88].

5.18. Let-7

Let-7 expression is not downregulated in human glioblastoma tissues and cell lines, let-7 ectopic overexpression by transfection on U251 and U87 human glioblastoma cells, reduced in vitro proliferation and migration and also in vivo tumor growth after xenotransplantation into nude mice. Furthermore, let-7 miRNA reduced the expression of total RAS, N-RAS, and K-RAS in glioblastoma cells [92]. These results suggest that let-7 miRNA is able to impair glioblastoma growth and cellular migration via RAS inhibition.

6. MicroRNAs and tumor stem cells

Glioma stem cells (GSCs) have been recently identified [93]. They express common neural stem cell (NSC) markers (CD133, Nestin, Musashi, and Sox2) and display multiple-lineage differentiation potential and a greater tumorigenic activity in rodent xenografts. GSCs also show an increased angiogenic potential through a higher expression of vascular endothelial growth factor (VEGF). GSCs are strongly resistant to radiation [94]and chemotherapy [95].

A recent study by Lavon et al showed a similar expression pattern of mir-21, mir-124, and mir-137 in gliomas and stem cells. Among them we mention the miR-17 family cluster that contains 3 miRNAs upregulated in gliomas and NPCs (mir-17-92, mir-106b-25, mir-106a); the mir-183-182 cluster, also upregulated in gliomas and NPCs; the large 7+46 bipartite miRNA cluster on chromosome 14, as most of miRNAs located within this region have been shown to be downregulated in the same samples [96]. This latter cluster is located within a region which shows a frequent loss of heterozygosity in glioblastomas [97]. Finally, mir302-367 cluster on chromosome 4q25 and mir371-373 cluster on chromosome 19q13, are upregulated in gliomas and NPCs. These data confirm the hypothesis that brain cancers arise from multipotent GSCs, thus explaining the phenotypic heterogeneity of tumors.

Many groups investigated the role of miRNAs in GSCs so far: in a first report Silber et al found that mir-124 and mir-137 are reduced in grade III and IV gliomas compared to normal brain. Besides, transfection of these two miRNAs in neural stem cells and glioma cancer cell lines leads to induction of cellular markers of differentiation, G1 cell cycle arrest and reductions of CDK6, thus indicating a hypothetical tumor suppressor role of micro-124 and microRNA-137 in GSCs [29]. As previously mentioned in this review, mir-128 was identified as a negative regulator of glioma self renewal when ectopically overexpressed on human glioma neurosphere cultures [58].

A recent analysis showed that mir-451 is significantly downregulated in CD133+cells. Transfection of miR-451 inhibits proliferation and neurosphere formation in GSCs, highlighting that it can act as a tumor suppressor: two target sites for SMAD protein in the upstream promoter region of miR-451 have been found, leading to draw the conclusion that this miRNA is activated by SMAD pathway. Transfection of SMAD in GBM cells inhibited their growth, suggesting it could induce differentiation of glioma CD133+stem cells through up-regulation of miR-451, thus reducing their tumorigenicity [98].In conclusion, a stable and selective delivery of these miRNAs to GSCs could represent a great advance for brain tumor therapy.

MiR -125b is required for stem cell fission, allowing them to bypass the G1/S checkpoint and making them insensitive to chemotherapy [99]. It has been found to be significantly downregulated in CD133+glioma stem cells compared to CD133-ones, leading to the hypothesis that it may be involved in cell differentiation. As expected, transfection of mir-125b to CD133+cells, decreased the number of proliferating cells and induced G0-G1 arrest: this effect occurs through a mir-125b-dependent downregulation of CDC25A and CDK6, two cell cycle regulatory proteins [47]. Moreover, miR-29b and miR-125a, are under-expressed in glioblastoma CD133+cells compared with their counterpart CD133-cells (see above), suggesting a potential role for these microRNAs in regulation of signaling pathways related to maintenance of stem cell properties and self-renewal of cancer cells [79].

Some miRNAs could have a role in the regulation of key pathways of GSCs. We already mentioned above the existence of a regulatory feedback loop between the tumor suppressor mir-326 and Notch pathway, shifted towards a prevalence of Notch activity in brain tumor cells and GSCs [80] Recently, pyruvate kinase type M2 (PKM2) has been identified as a putative target of mir-326, as levels of PKM2 and mir-326 are inversely correlated in glioma cells. PKM2, highly expressed on cancer cells and GSCs, plays the role of mediator in mir-326 metabolic effects: experimental knockdown of this molecule led to an impairment of glioma invasiveness and clonogenicity and decreased ATP levels, suggesting that PKM2 could represent a valid target for glioma therapy [100].

Mir-34a downregulated in gliomas and GSCs. When transfected into GSCs, it decreased the expression of the stem cell markers CD133 and nestin and caused an higher immunostaining for astrocytes and oligodendrocytes markers, besides modestly inhibiting several malignancy end-points (migration, survival, proliferation, cell cycle progression). Remarkably, miR-34a levels in glioma stem cells are significantly lower than in differentiated wild-type p53 glioma cell lines, suggesting that restoration of miR-34a expression for therapeutic purposes could achieve strong anti-tumor effects not only by targeting differentiated glioma cells, but also by inducing glioma stem cell differentiation [56].

7. MicroRNAs in medulloblastoma

Medulloblastoma (MB) is the most common brain malignancy observed in childhood (WHO grade IV) [101]. Ferretti et al were the first showed that miRNAs profiles is different between primary medulloblastomas and normal cerebellar controls. These aberrant miRNAs have a potentially role in MB development: e.g., let-7 microRNAs has been shown to inhibit Ras oncogene expression [102], reported to be a key factor for MB metastatic behavior [103]; miR-17-92 cluster cooperates with myc, frequently overexpressed in MB, to induce neoplastic transformation [104]; miR-9 and miR-125a, both downregulated in MB, are involved in cell proliferation and, when transfected into MB cells, promote apoptosis and impair anchorage-independent growth by downregulating the truncated isoform of the neurotropin receptor TrkC (t-TrkC). T-TrkC expression levels are higher in MB, inversely correlate with miR-9 and miR-125a levels and are responsible of enhanced cell proliferation and worse prognosis. Mir-9 and mir-124 have a common molecular target, REST/NRSF (RE1 silencing transcription factor/ neuron-restrictive silencer factor) complex [105]. These observations suggest that Mir-9 and mir-124 could play an important role in cerebellar tumorigenesis as REST inactivation has been reported to inhibit tumor growth [106] and is overexpressed in many MBs [107]. Consequently, a REST/mir-124 axis shifted towards a prevalence of REST activity, could block neuronal differen-tiation and promote neoplastic transformation [108].

Mir-124 also modulates medulloblastoma growth by targeting CDK6, a key pro-proliferative factor overexpressed in 30% of medulloblastomas, which represents an adverse prognostic marker for clinical outcome [109]. The role of mir-124 in MB development was later confirmed by Li et al who additionally demonstrated that ectopic expression of mir-124 in medulloblas-toma cell lines inhibits cell growth by directly targeting SLC16A1, a protein upregulated in MBs, that serve as a carrier to export lactic acid extracellularly, thus maintaining homeostasis of tumor cells, where aerobic glycolysis is known to be accelerated [110].At the same time, downregulation of miR-218 could account for an overexpression of the pro-oncogene EGFR, which activates MAPK pathway and CTNND2, which in turn encodes the gene of β-catenin that activates the APC/Wnt signal transduction pathway and leads to tumor growth [111].

Hedgehog (Hh) patched (Ptch1) signalling pathway is a key regulator of the development of cerebellar granule cell progenitors and its constitutive activation makes cells susceptible of malignant transformation into medulloblastoma [112]. Hh is a secreted protein that binds to the transmembrane receptor Ptch1 transducing an intracellular signal through the protoon-cogene Smoothened (Smo) to the downstream transcription factors Gli1, Gli2, and Gli3 [113].

Ferretti et al found that miR-125b, miR-326 and miR-324-5p target and repress activator downstream components of the Hh signalling pathway (Smo and Gli1); consistent with these findings, 50% of MBs showed a downregulation of these miRNAs together with an overex-pression of Gli1. Deletion of chromosome 17p, the most frequent mutation in medulloblasto-ma, could account for several genetic defects, including miR-324-5p, p53 and HIC1 tumor suppressors loss, which cooperate in Hh-dependent tumorigenesis: loss of these genes, together with other molecular events, contribute to a persistent hyperactivation of Hh signalling during cerebellar granule cell progenitors development, leading to higher prolifer-ative activity and susceptibility to malignant MBs [114].

Recently, Hedgehog signalling pathway has been identified as a target of miR-17-92 cluster. Indeed, miRNAs from the miR-17-92 cluster are specifically overexpressed in mouse MB models with specific initiating mutations in Ptch1 and in human MB subgroups with an activated SHH signaling pathway. To evaluate its oncogenic potential, miR-17-92 was retrovirally transduced into mouse granule neuron progenitors cells (GNPs) before orthotopic transplantation into immunocompromised mice. Interestingly, only cells with an SHH signaling defect (Ptc+/-) developed MBs. Tumor cells from this model exhibited markers of activated SHH signaling as elevated Math1 and Gli1 mRNA levels, and lost expression of the wild-type Ptc allele, reinforcing the hypothesis of a functional link between the SHH pathway and this miRNA cluster [115]. Some studies showed that miR-17-92 is most highly expressed in SHH-driven medulloblastomas, and higher levels of miR-17-92 are also related to an overexpression of the oncogene MYC. Moreover, transfection of miR-17-92 maintains mouse CGNP cells in a proliferative state in the absence of SHH, and synergizes with SHH to promote cell growth, while treatment of the same cells with SHH results in upregulation of miR-17-92, confirming that this cooperation is crucial in MB tumorigenesis [116].

Notch pathway plays a key role in regulating granule-cell progenitor differentiation and an increased copy number of Notch-2 was detected in 15% of medulloblastomas [117]. Expression of the downstream effector of Notch, HES1, normally declines during neuronal differentiation, while persistent activation of this factor prevents differentiation of precursor cells [118]. Garzia et al identified mir-199-5p as capable of directly targeting and repress expression of HES1 in MB cell lines. Ectopic expression of this miRNA reduced MB cell proliferation, population expressing stem cell marker CD133 and xenograft tumor growth in mouse models. Their studies also suggest that the documented downregulation of miR-199b-5p in metastatic tumors may be related to epigenetic silencing [119].

Venkataraman et al recently showed that several miRNAs known to be involved in CNS development, are downregulated in medulloblastoma cell line cultures and tissues. A specific one, miR-128a, is able to decrease tumor growth and proliferation if ectopically re-expressed on MB cells. Bmi-1 has been identified as a putative target of miR-128a, a critical factor in cerebellar development frequently upregulated in MBs. MiR-128a seems to normally down-regulate Bmi-1 oncogene, leading to increased levels of p16, a cell cycle inhibitor. Furthermore, Bmi-1 could be involved in regulating reactive oxygen species by decreasing superoxide generation, thus leading to a lower redox state in cancer stem cells [120]; this event is known to be partially responsible of tumor resistance against common therapies [121].

Finally, mir-34a appeared to be a tumor suppressor gene also in medulloblastomas other than in glioblastomas. Indeed, transient transfection of miR-34a into medulloblastoma cell lines, strongly inhibited cell proliferation, cell cycle progression, cell survival and cell invasion most probably through a direct inhibition of c-Met [56].

8. MiRNAs in pituitary tumors

Pituitary adenomas are benign and frequent neoplasms, accounting for about 15% of primary intracranial tumors [122]. Bottoni et al found that 30 miRNAs are differentially expressed between normal pituitary gland and pituitary adenomas. Furthermore, their expression is inversely correlated with tumor size. They probably act through a negative regulation of RARS (arginyl-tRNA synthetase), which is in turn upregulated in pituitary adenomas and modulates the expression of factors influencing pituitary tumor growth [123]. Mir-15a and mir-16-1 are located within chromosome region 13q14. Interestingly, loss of 13q region of chromosome 13 was frequently detected in pituitary tumors, confirming that this region likely contains tumor suppressor genes [124].

These findings support the hypothesis that miRNA-16-1 plays a key role in tumor growth [195], most probably by interacting with BCL2 [125], which is overexpressed in about one third of pituitary adenomas [126]. MiRNAome could also function as a signature for specific histotypes of pituitary adenomas. Overexpression of miR-23a, miR-23b, and miR-24-2 and lower expression of mir-26b are more typical of GH-secreting and PRL-secreting adenomas, differentiating them from non-functioning adenomas (NFA), characterized by mir-26 upregulation and miRNA-24-2 downregulation. Moreover, NFA express higher concentration of miR-137 and lower of miR-127, miR-129, miR-203, and miR-134 compared to GH-secreting adenomas. Finally, ACTH-secreting adenomas are defined by a strong expression of mir-30 cluster (miR-30a, miR-30b, miR-30c, and miR-30d), supporting the hypothesis that miRNAs could be useful diagnostic markers to distinguish pituitary tumor histotypes [127].More recently, Amaral et al evaluated the expression of microRNAs in ACTH-secreting pituitary tumors: they found that let-7a, miR-21, miR-141, miR-143, miR-145, and miR-150, besides miR-15 and miR-16, are downregulated in corticotropinomas compared to normal pituitary tissue and that a lower expression of mir-141 is linked to a better chance of remission after surgery [128]. Moreover, downregulation of Mir-143 could be involved in tumorigenesis by activating MAPK pathway via ERK5 [129].

Quian et al showed that let-7 expression is decreased in more than one third of pituitary adenomas and is related to higher tumor grade, thus it may act as a tumor suppressor. Levels of let-7 were found to be inversely correlated to HMGA2 expression [130], confirming some previous studies which showed that HMGA2 is repressed by let-7 [131]. High levels of HMGA2 have been detected in most types of pituitary adenomas [132] and they are significantly associated with tumor grade, extent of invasion, tumor size and Ki-67 proliferation index, probably through regulation of E-cadherin, E2F1, cyclin A, and p53 expression. Accordingly, let-7 may be useful as a novel anticancer agent in the future [130]. A recent study on the role of miRNAs in NFAs and GH-secreting pituitary tumors was performed by Butz et al, showing that a group of miRNAs (miR-128a, miR-155, and miR-516a-3p) targets the 3'-untranslated region of Wee1, a nuclear protein kinase that acts as a tumor suppressor, and which was found to be significantly decreased in pituitary tumor samples [133].

9. Therapeutic potential of miRNAs

Current evidence indicates that miRNA deregulation is common in human cancers. The discovery of miRNAs with oncogenic or tumor-suppressive function raises the possibility of exploiting these RNA molecules for therapeutic intervention and the development of novel therapies. The oncogenic miRNAs can be downregulated using antisense miRNA oligonu-cleotides (AMOs or antagomirs) or miRNA sponges[134,135], whereas tumor-suppressive miRNAs may be targeted by replacement with miRNA mimetics.

AMOs are synthetic oligonucleotides with sequence complementary either to mature miRNA or its precursor and have been widely used to inhibit miRNA activities in vitro and in vivo[136]. A number of chemical modifications to AMOs have been developed to improve specific binding to target miRNAs and to resist nuclease degradation. These in-clude modifications at the 20-hydroxyl position (20-O-methyl (20OMe), 20-Omethoxyeth-yl(20MOE), 20-fluoro (20F) and locked nucleic acids (LNA)), on the phosphorothioate backbone, and conjugation with cholesterol [137]. Of these modifications,LNA shows high stability, strong affinity for target miRNAs and low toxicity in biological system and has emerged as a strong candidate for targeting miRNAs in vivo. One clinical trial using LNA anti-miRNA in treating human disease has been initiated recently. Using LNA antimiR-21, Corsten et al. demonstrated that miR-21 knockdown in glioma cells led to an increase of apoptotic cell death and a significant reduction of glioma growth in vivo, suggesting that miR-21 is a potential therapeutic target. They further showed that combination of miR-21 suppression and the cytotoxic agent tumor necrosis factor-related apoptosis-inducing ligand (TRAIL) resulted in enhanced caspase activity and synergistic killing of glioma cells in vitro. When these treated glioma cells were implanted intracra-nially into nude mice, tumor cells were completely eradicated after day 6 of implanta-tion, compared to reduced tumor volume with either treatment alone. This finding suggests that miR-21 knockdown sensitizes glioma cells to apoptosis agent, and that the combined treatment is a promising approach for glioma elimination [138].

Angiogenesis is a process essential for malignant glioma growth. By co-culturing glioma cells with microvascular endothelial cells, Wurdinger et al. showed that glioma cells could induce changes of miRNA expression in endothelial cells, with miR-296 being significantly upregulated. Enhanced expression of miR-296 was also observed in endothelial cells treated with glioma-conditioned medium or proangiogenic growth factor VEGF or EGF, as well as in endothelial cells isolated from glioma samples. These results suggested a role for miR-296 in angiogenesis. It was further demonstrated that miR-296 contributed to angiogenesis by targeting hepatocyte growth factor-regulated tyrosine kinase substrate (HGS), which controls the levels of growth factor receptors (VEGFR2 and PDGFRb) by directing these macromolecules to lysosomes for degradation. Importantly, intravenous administration of antimiR- 296 AMO significantly reduced angiogenesis in glioma xenografts in vivo[139]. These results suggest that inhibition of angiogenesis by targeting miR-296 in endothelial cells may represent an alternative approach in glioma therapy.

10. Conclusion

MiRNAs are an astonishing new class of gene regulators, and it had been demonstrated that these molecules play a crucial role in cancer development and progression in a variety of malignancies, including brain tumors. Most importantly, in a clinical context, there is first evidence that miRNAs might provide new options to improve diagnostics and therapy in the two most common malignant primary brain tumors in adults (glioblastoma) and children (medulloblastoma). In vitro and in vivo data suggest that miRNAs could be used to discriminate brain tumors from normal brain tissue, and to identify different astrocytoma grades. More important, clinico-pathological features seem to correlate with miRNA expression in these tumors. Furthermore, there is increasing evidence that miRNAs might help to generate targeted therapies and to overcome resistance to conventional anticancer strategies for example in glioblastomas. Of course, it has to be acknowledged at this stage that translation of these preliminary "in vitro data" into "hard clinical facts" is not feasible. But these findings provide a very promising basis for future studies to determine the effect of miRNA modulation on chemotherapy in "in vivo studies". Although therapeutic delivery of miRNAs is still a developing field, and there is much more work to be done before these molecules can be securely applied in clinical settings, miRNA modulation may one day have a therapeutic application in patients. In summary, the presented data supports the enormous clinical potential of miRNAs in brain tumors, and mandate further intensive investigations in this field.

Acknowledgements

Supported by China National Natural Scientific Found (30901772).

Author details

Chunzhi Zhang[1], Budong Chen[2], Xiangying Xu[3], Baolin Han[3], Guangshun Wang[3] and Jinhuan Wang[2]

1 Department of Radiation Oncology, Tianjin Huan Hu Hospital, Tianjin, China

2 Department of Neurosurgery, Tianjin Huan Hu Hospital, Tianjin, China

3 Department of Oncology, Tianjin Baodi Hospital, Tianjin, China

References

[1] Feng, W, & Feng, Y. MicroRNAs in neural cell development and brain diseases. Sci China Life Sci. (2011).

[2] Zen, K, & Zhang, C. Y. Circulating MicroRNAs: a novel class of biomarkers to diagnose and monitor human cancers. Med Res Rev. (2012).

[3] Rottiers, V, & Näär, A. M. MicroRNAs in metabolism and metabolic disorders. Nat Rev Mol Cell Biol. (2012).

[4] Babashah, S, & Soleimani, M. The oncogenic and tumour suppressive roles of microRNAs in cancer and apoptosis. Eur J Cancer. (2011).

[5] Calin, G. A, Sevignani, C, Dumitru, C. D, Hyslop, T, Noch, E, Yendamuri, S, Shimizu, M, Rattan, S, Bullrich, F, Negrini, M, & Croce, C. M. Human microRNA genes are frequently located at fragile sites and genomic regions involved in cancers. Proc Natl Acad Sci USA.(2004).

[6] Lu, J, Getz, G, Miska, E. A, Alvarez-saavedra, E, Lamb, J, Peck, D, Sweet-cordero, A, Ebert, B. L, Mak, R. H, Ferrando, A. A, Downing, J. R, Jacks, T, Horvitz, H. R, & Golub, T. R. MicroRNA expression profiles classify human cancers. Nature.(2005).

[7] Volinia, S, Calin, G. A, Liu, C. G, Ambs, S, Cimmino, A, Petrocca, F, Visone, R, Iorio, M, Roldo, C, Ferracin, M, Prueitt, R. L, Yanaihara, N, Lanza, G, Scarpa, A, Vecchione, A, Negrini, M, Harris, C. C, & Croce, C. M. A microRNA expression signature of human solid tumors defines cancer gene targets. Proc Natl Acad Sci USA.(2006).

[8] Bottoni, A, Piccin, D, Tagliati, F, Luchin, A, & Zatelli, M. C. degliUberti EC. miR-15a and miR-down-regulation in pituitary adenomas. J Cell Physiol.(2005). , 16-1.

[9] Chan, J. A, Krichevsky, A. M, & Kosik, K. S. MicroRNA-21 is an antiapoptotic factor in human glioblastoma cells. Cancer Res.(2005).

[10] Ciafrè, S. A, Galardi, S, Mangiola, A, Ferracin, M, Liu, C. G, Sabatino, G, Negrini, M, Maira, G, Croce, C. M, & Farace, M. G. Extensive modulation of a set of microRNAs in primary glioblastoma. Biochem Biophys Res Commun.(2005).

[11] Sasayama, T, Nishihara, M, Kondoh, T, Hosoda, K, & Kohmura, E. MicroRNA-10b is overexpressed in malignant glioma and associated with tumor invasive factors, uP-AR and RhoC. Int J Cancer.(2009).

[12] Xia, H, Qi, Y, Ng, S. S, Chen, X, Li, D, Chen, S, Ge, R, Jiang, S, Li, G, Chen, Y, He, M. L, Kung, H. F, Lai, L, & Lin, M. C. microRNA-146b inhibits glioma cell migration and invasion by targeting MMPs. Brain Res.(2009).

[13] Cortez, M. A, Nicoloso, M. S, Shimizu, M, Rossi, S, Gopisetty, G, & Molina, J. R. Carlotti C Jr, Tirapelli D, Neder L, Brassesco MS, Scrideli CA, Tone LG, Georgescu MM, Zhang W, Puduvalli V, Calin GA. miR-29b and miR-125a regulate podoplanin and suppress invasion in glioblastoma. Genes Chromosomes Cancer.(2010).

[14] Silber, J, Lim, DA, Petritsch, C, Persson, AI, Maunakea, AK, Yu, M, Vandenberg, SR, Ginzinger, DG, James, CD, Costello, JF, Bergers, G, Weiss, WA, Alvarez-Buylla, A, Hodgson, JG, & mi, . -137 inhibit proliferation of glioblastoma multiforme cells and induce differentiation of brain tumor stem cells. BMC Med.2008, 6:14

[15] Rao, S. A, Santosh, V, & Somasundaram, K. Genome-wide expression profiling identifies deregulated miRNAs in malignant astrocytoma. Mod Pathol. (2010).

[16] Ferretti, E, De Smaele, E, & Po, A. Di Marcotullio L, Tosi E, Espinola MS, Di Rocco C, Riccardi R, Giangaspero F, Farcomeni A, Nofroni I, Laneve P, Gioia U, Caffarelli E, Bozzoni I, Screpanti I, Gulino A. MicroRNA profiling in human medulloblastoma. Int J Cancer. (2009).

[17] Bottoni, A, Zatelli, M. C, Ferracin, M, Tagliati, F, Piccin, D, Vignali, C, Calin, G. A, Negrini, M, & Croce, C. M. Degli Uberti EC. Identification of differentially expressed microRNAs by microarray: a possible role for microRNA genes in pituitary adenomas. J Cell Physiol. (2007).

[18] Zhi, F, Zhou, G, Wang, S, Shi, Y, Peng, Y, Shao, N, Guan, W, Qu, H, Zhang, Y, Wang, Q, Yang, C, Wang, R, Wu, S, Xia, X, & Yang, Y. A microRNA expression signature predicts meningioma recurrence. Int J Cancer. (2012). doi:ijc.27658.

[19] Niyazi, M, Zehentmayr, F, Niemöller, O. M, Eigenbrod, S, Kretzschmar, H, Schulze-osthoff, K, Tonn, J. C, Atkinson, M, Mörtl, S, & Belka, C. MiRNA expression patterns predict survival in glioblastoma. Radiat Oncol. (2011).

[20] Ma, R, Yan, W, Zhang, G, Lv, H, Liu, Z, Fang, F, Zhang, W, Zhang, J, Tao, T, You, Y, Jiang, T, & Kang, X. Upregulation of miR-196b Confers a Poor Prognosis in Glioblastoma Patients via Inducing a Proliferative Phenotype. PLoS One. (2012). e38096.

[21] Costa, F. F, Bischof, J. M, Vanin, E. F, Lulla, R. R, Wang, M, Sredni, S. T, & Rajaram, V. Bonaldo Mde F, Wang D, Goldman S, Tomita T, Soares MB. Identification of microRNAs as potential prognostic markers in ependymoma. PLoS One. (2011). e25114.

[22] Liu, J, Zheng, M, Tang, Y. L, Liang, X. H, & Yang, Q. MicroRNAs, an active and versatile group in cancers. Int J Oral Sci. (2011).

[23] Calin, G. A, Dumitru, C. D, Shimizu, M, Bichi, R, Zupo, S, Noch, E, Aldler, H, Rattan, S, Keating, M, Rai, K, Rassenti, L, Kipps, T, Negrini, M, Bullrich, F, & Croce, C. M. Frequent deletions and down-regulation of micro- RNA genes miR15 and miR16 at 13q14 in chronic lymphocytic leukemia.Proc Natl Acad Sci U S A. (2002).

[24] Cimmino, A, Calin, GA, Fabbri, M, Iorio, MV, Ferracin, M, Shimizu, M, Wojcik, SE, Aqeilan, RI, Zupo, S, Dono, M, Rassenti, L, Alder, H, Volinia, S, Liu, CG, Kipps, TJ, Negrini, M, Croce, CM, & mi, . -16 induce apoptosis by targeting BCL2.Proc Natl Acad Sci U S A. 2005,102(39):13944-13949.

[25] Mu, P, Han, Y. C, Betel, D, Yao, E, Squatrito, M, Ogrodowski, P, De Stanchina, E, Andrea, D, Sander, A, & Ventura, C. A. Genetic dissection of the miR-17~92 cluster of microRNAs in Myc-induced B-cell lymphomas. Genes Dev. (2009).

[26] Zhang ChunzhiKang Chunsheng, You Yongpin, Pu Peiyu, Yang Weidong, Zhao Peng, Wang Guangxiu, Zhang Anling, Jia Zhifan, Han Lei and Jiang Hao. Co-suppression of miR-221/222 cluster suppresses human glioma cells growth by targeting in vitro and in vivo. International Journal of Oncology.(2009). , 27kip1.

[27] Chun-Zhi ZhangJun-Xia Zhang, An-Ling Zhang, Zhen-Dong Shi, Lei Han, Zhi-Fan Jia, Wei-Dong Yang, Guang-Xiu Wang, Tao Jiang, Yong-Ping You, Pei-Yu Pu, Jin-Quan Cheng, Chun-Sheng Kang. MiR-221 and miR-222 target PUMA to induce Cell suvivall in glioblastoma. Molecular Cancer. (2010).

[28] Zhang, C, Zhang, J, Hao, J, Shi, Z, Wang, Y, Han, L, Yu, S, You, Y, Jiang, T, Wang, J, Liu, M, Pu, P, & Kang, C. High level of miR-221/222 confers increased cell invasion and poor prognosis in glioma. J Transl Med. (2012).

[29] Niemoeller, O. M, Niyazi, M, Corradini, S, Zehentmayr, F, Li, M, Lauber, K, & Belka, G. MicroRNA expression profiles in human cancer cells after ionizing radiation. Radiat. Oncol. (2011).

[30] Chistiakov, D. A, & Chekhonin, V. P. Contribution of microRNAs to radio- and chemoresistance of brain tumors and their therapeutic potential. Eur J Pharmacol. (2012).

[31] Wild-bode, C, Weller, M, Rimner, A, Dichgans, J, & Wick, W. Sublethal irradiation promotes migration and invasiveness of glioma cells: implications for radiotherapy of human glioblastoma. Cancer Res. (2001).

[32] Medina, R, Zaidi, S. K, Liu, C. G, Stein, J. L, Van Wijnen, A. J, Croce, C. M, & Stein, G. S. MicroRNAs 221 and 222 bypass quiescence and compromise cell survival. Cancer Res.(2008).

[33] Zhang, C, Kang, C, Wang, P, Cao, Y, Lv, Z, Yu, S, Wang, G, Zhang, A, Jia, Z, Han, L, Yang, C, Ishiyama, H, Teh, B. S, Xu, B, & Pu, P. MicroRNA-221/-222 regulate radiation sensitivity by targeting the PTEN pathway. Int J Radiat Oncol Biol Phys, (2011).

[34] Hao, J, Zhang, C, Zhang, A, Wang, K, Jia, Z, Wang, G, Han, L, Kang, C, Pu, P, & mi, . -221/222 is the regulator of Cx43 expression in human glioblastoma cells. Oncol Rep, 2012,27(5): 1504-1510.

[35] Chan, J. A, Krichevsky, A. M, & Kosik, K. S. MicroRNA-21 is an antiapoptotic factor in human glioblastoma cells. Cancer Res.(2005).

[36] Conti, A, & Aguennouz, M. La Torre D, Tomasello C, Cardali S, Angileri FF, Maio F, Cama A, Germanò A, Vita G and Tomasello F. miR-21 and 221 upregulation and miR-181b downregulation in human grade II-IV astrocytic tumors. J Neurooncol. (2009).

[37] Zhi, F, Chen, X, Wang, S, Xia, X, Shi, Y, Guan, W, Shao, N, Qu, H, Yang, C, Zhang, Y, Wang, Q, Wang, R, Zen, K, Zhang, C. Y, Zhang, J, & Yang, Y. The use of hsa-miR-21, hsa-miR-181b and hsa-miR-106a as prognostic indicators of astrocytoma. Eur J Cancer.(2010).

[38] Corsten, M. F, Miranda, R, Kasmieh, R, Krichevsky, A. M, Weissleder, R, & Shah, K. MicroRNA-21 knockdown disrupts glioma growth in vivo and displays synergistic cytotoxicity with neural precursor cell delivered S-TRAIL in human gliomas. Cancer Res.(2007).

[39] Zhou, X, Zhang, J, Jia, Q, Ren, Y, Wang, Y, Shi, L, Liu, N, Wang, G, Pu, P, You, Y, & Kang, C. Reduction of miR-21 induces glioma cell apoptosis via activating caspase 9 and 3. Oncol Rep.(2010).

[40] Shi, L, Cheng, Z, Zhang, J, Li, R, You, Y, & Fu, Z. The mechanism of apoptosis in human U87 glioma cells induced by miR-21 antisense oligonucleotide. Zhonghua Yi Xue Yi Chuan Xue Za Zhi.(2008).

[41] Papagiannakopoulos, T, Shapiro, A, & Kosik, K. S. MicroRNA-21 targets a network of key tumor-suppressive pathways in glioblastoma cells. Cancer Res.(2008).

[42] Chen, Y, Liu, W, Chao, T, Zhang, Y, Yan, X, Gong, Y, Qiang, B, Yuan, J, Sun, M, & Peng, X. MicroRNA-21 down-regulates the expression of tumor suppressor PDCD4 in human glioblastoma cell T98G. Cancer Lett.(2008).

[43] Gabriely, G, Wurdinger, T, Kesari, S, Esau, C. C, Burchard, J, Linsley, P. S, & Krichevsky, A. M. MicroRNA 21 promotes glioma invasion by targeting matrix metalloproteinase regulators. Mol Cell Biol.(2008).

[44] Endersby, R, & Baker, S. J. PTEN signaling in brain: neuropathology and tumorigenesis. Oncogene.(2008).

[45] Leslie, N. R, & Downes, C. P. PTEN: The down side of PI kinase signalling. Cell Signal.(2002). , 3.

[46] Zhou, X, Ren, Y, Moore, L, Mei, M, You, Y, Xu, P, Wang, B, Wang, G, Jia, Z, Pu, P, Zhang, W, & Kang, C. Downregulation of miR-21 inhibits EGFR pathway and suppresses the growth of human glioblastoma cells independent of PTEN status. Lab Invest.(2010).

[47] Shi, L, Chen, J, Yang, J, Pan, T, Zhang, S, Wang, Z, & Mi, . -21 protected human glioblastoma U87MG cells from chemotherapeutic drug temozolomide induced apoptosis by decreasing Bax/Bcl-2 ratio and caspase-3 activity. Brain Res.2010, 1352: 255-264.

[48] Li, Y, Li, W, Yang, Y, Lu, Y, He, C, Hu, G, Liu, H, Chen, J, He, J, & Yu, H. MicroRNA-21 targets LRRFIP1 and contributes to VM-26 resistance in glioblastoma multiforme. Brain Res.(2009).

[49] Lee, S. Y, Lee, S. Y, & Choi, Y. TRAF-interacting protein (TRIP): a novel component of the tumor necrosis factor receptor (TNFR)- and CDTRAF signaling complexes that inhibits TRAF2-mediated NF-kappaB activation. J Exp Med.(1997). , 30.

[50] Nakanishi, C, & Toi, M. Nuclear factor-kappaB inhibitors as sensitizers to anticancer drugs. Nat Rev Cancer. (2005).

[51] Ren, Y, Kang, C. S, Yuan, X. B, Zhou, X, Xu, P, Han, L, Wang, G. X, Jia, Z, Zhong, Y, Yu, S, Sheng, J, & Pu, P. Y. Co-delivery of as-miR-21 and FU by poly(amidoamine) dendrimer attenuates human glioma cell growth in vitro. J Biomater Sci Polym Ed. (2010). , 5.

[52] Ohno, M, Natsume, A, Kondo, Y, Iwamizu, H, Motomura, K, Toda, H, Ito, M, Kato, T, & Wakabayashi, T. The modulation of microRNAs by type I IFN through the activation of signal transducers and activators of transcription 3 in human glioma. Mol Cancer Res.(2009).

[53] Li, Y, Guessous, F, Zhang, Y, Dipierro, C, Kefas, B, Johnson, E, Marcinkiewicz, L, Jiang, J, Yang, Y, Schmittgen, T. D, Lopes, B, Schiff, D, Purow, B, & Abounader, R. MicroRNA-34a inhibits glioblastoma growth by targeting multiple oncogenes. Cancer Res.(2009).

[54] Luan, S, Sun, L, & Huang, F. MicroRNA-34a: a novel tumor suppressor in glioma cell line U251. Arch Med Res.(2010). , 53.

[55] Guessous, F, Zhang, Y, Kofman, A, Catania, A, Li, Y, Schiff, D, Purow, B, & Abounader, R. icroRNA-34a is tumor suppressive in brain tumors and glioma stem cells. Cell Cycle.(2010).

[56] Yan, D, Zhou, X, Chen, X, Hu, D. N, Dong, X. D, Wang, J, Lu, F, Tu, L, & Qu, J. MicroRNA-34a inhibits uveal melanoma cell proliferation and migration through downregulation of c-Met. Invest Ophthalmol Vis Sci.(2009).

[57] Huffman, D. M, Grizzle, W. E, Bamman, M. M, Kim, J. S, Eltoum, I. A, Elgavish, A, & Nagy, T. R. SIRT1 is significantly elevated in mouse and human prostate cancer. Cancer Res.(2007).

[58] Godlewski, J, Nowicki, M. O, Bronisz, A, Williams, S, Otsuki, A, Nuovo, G, Raychaudhury, A, Newton, H. B, Chiocca, E. A, & Lawler, S. Targeting of the Bmi-1 oncogene/stem cell renewal factor by microRNA-128 inhibits glioma proliferation and self-renewal. Cancer Res.(2008).

[59] Cui, J. G, Zhao, Y, Sethi, P, Li, Y. Y, Mahta, A, Culicchia, F, & Lukiw, W. J. MicroRNA-128 (miRNA-128) down-regulation in glioblastoma targets ARP5 (ANGPTL6), Bmi-1 and E2F-3a, key regulators of brain cell proliferation. J Neurooncol. (2010).

[60] Fasano, C. A, Dimos, J. T, Ivanova, N. B, Lowry, N, Lemischka, I. R, & Temple, S. shRNA knockdown of Bmi-1 reveals a critical role for pathway in NSC self-renewal during development. Cell Stem Cell. (2007). , 21.

[61] Guo, W. J, Zeng, M. S, Yadav, A, Song, L. B, Guo, B. H, Band, V, & Dimri, G. P. Mel-18 acts as a tumor suppressor by repressing Bmi-1 expression and down-regulating Akt activity in breast cancer cells. Cancer Res. (2007).

[62] Iaquinta, P. J, & Lees, J. A. Life and death decisions by the E2F transcription factors. Curr Opin Cell Biol. (2007).

[63] Oike, Y, Yasunaga, K, Ito, Y, Matsumoto, S, Maekawa, H, Morisada, T, Arai, F, Nakagata, N, Takeya, M, Masuho, Y, & Suda, T. Angiopoietin-related growth factor (AGF) promotes epidermal proliferation, remodeling, and regeneration. Proc Natl Acad Sci U S A. (2003).

[64] Huse, J. T, Brennan, C, Hambardzumyan, D, Wee, B, Pena, J, Rouhanifard, S. H, & Sohn-lee, C. Le Sage C, Agami R, Tuschl T and Holland EC. The PTEN-regulating microRNA miR-26a is amplified in high-grade glioma and facilitates gliomagenesis in vivo. Genes Dev. (2009).

[65] Godlewski, J, Nowicki, M. O, Bronisz, A, & Nuovo, G. Palatini JDe Lay M, Van Brocklyn J, Ostrowski MC, Chiocca EA andLawler SE. MicroRNA-451 regulates LKB1/AMPK signalingand allows adaptation to metabolic stress in glioma cells. Mol Cell. (2010).

[66] Alessi, D. R, Sakamoto, K, & Bayascas, J. R. LKB1-dependent signaling pathways. Annu Rev Biochem.(2006). , 75, 137-163.

[67] Nan, Y, Han, L, Zhang, A, Wang, G, Jia, Z, Yang, Y, Yue, X, Pu, P, Zhong, Y, & Kang, C. MiRNA-451 plays a role as tumor suppressor in human glioma cells. Brain Res. (2010).

[68] Kefas, B, Godlewski, J, Comeau, L, Li, Y, Abounader, R, Hawkinson, M, Lee, J, Fine, H, Chiocca, E. A, Lawler, S, & Purow, B. microRNA-7 inhibits the epidermal growth

factor receptor and the Akt pathway and is down-regulated in glioblastoma. Cancer Res. (2008).

[69] Webster, R. J, Giles, K. M, Price, K. J, Zhang, P. M, Mattick, J. S, & Leedman, P. J. Regulation of epidermal growth factor receptor signaling in human cancer cells by microRNA-7. J Biol Chem. (2009).

[70] Reddy, S. D, Ohshiro, K, Rayala, S. K, & Kumar, R. MicroRNA-7, a homeobox D10 target, inhibits kinase 1 and regulates its functions. Cancer Res. (2008). , 21.

[71] Kumar, R, Gururaj, A. E, & Barnes, C. J. p. activated kinases in cancer. Nat Rev Cancer. (2006). , 21.

[72] Aoki, H, Yokoyama, T, Fujiwara, K, Tari, A. M, Sawaya, R, Suki, D, Hess, K. R, Aldape, K. D, Kondo, S, Kumar, R, & Kondo, Y. Phosphorylated Pak1 level in the cytoplasm correlates with shorter survival time in patients with glioblastoma. Clin Cancer Res. (2007). Pt 1):6603-6609.

[73] Miska, E. A, Alvarez-saavedra, E, Townsend, M, Yoshii, A, Sestan, N, Rakic, P, Constantine-paton, M, & Horvitz, H. R. Microarray analysis of microRNA expression in the developing mammalian brain. Genome Biol. (2004). R68.

[74] Shi, L, Cheng, Z, Zhang, J, Li, R, Zhao, P, Fu, Z, You, Y, & Hsa-mir, a. and hsa-mir-181b function as tumor suppressors in human glioma cells. Brain Res. (2008).

[75] Slaby, O, Lakomy, R, Fadrus, P, Hrstka, R, Kren, L, Lzicarova, E, Smrcka, M, Svoboda, M, Dolezalova, H, Novakova, J, Valik, D, Vyzula, R, & Michalek, J. MicroRNA-181 family predicts response to concomitant chemoradiotherapy with temozolomide in glioblastoma patients. Neoplasma. (2010).

[76] Silber, J, Lim, DA, Petritsch, C, Persson, AI, Maunakea, AK, Yu, M, Vandenberg, SR, Ginzinger, DG, James, CD, Costello, JF, Bergers, G, Weiss, WA, Alvarez-Buylla, A, Hodgson, JG, & mi, . -137 inhibit proliferation of glioblastoma multiforme cells and induce differentiation of brain tumor stem cells. BMC Med. 2008,6:14.

[77] Xia, HF, He, TZ, Liu, CM, Cui, Y, Song, PP, Jin, XH, Ma, X, & Mi, . -125b expression affects the proliferation and apoptosis of human glioma cells by targeting Bmf. Cell Physiol Biochem. 2009;23(4-6):347-358.

[78] Puthalakath, H, Villunger, A, Reilly, O, Beaumont, L. A, Coultas, J. G, Cheney, L, Huang, R. E, Strasser, D. C, Bmf, A, & Proapoptotic, a. BHonly protein regulated by interaction with the myosin V actin motor complex, activated by anoikis. Science. (2001). , 3.

[79] Cortez, M. A, Nicoloso, M. S, Shimizu, M, Rossi, S, Gopisetty, G, & Molina, J. R. Carlotti C Jr, Tirapelli D, Neder L, Brassesco MS, Scrideli CA, Tone LG, Georgescu MM, Zhang W, Puduvalli V, Calin GA. miR-29b and miR-125a regulate podoplanin and suppress invasion in glioblastoma. Genes Chromosomes Cancer. (2010).

[80] Kefas, B, Comeau, L, Floyd, D. H, Seleverstov, O, Godlewski, J, Schmittgen, T, & Jiang, J. diPierro CG, Li Y, Chiocca EA, Lee J, Fine H, Abounader R, Lawler S, Purow B. The neuronal microRNA miR-326 acts in a feedback loop with notch and has therapeutic potential against brain tumors. J Neurosci. (2009).

[81] Kim, H, Huang, W, Jiang, X, Pennicooke, B, Park, P. J, & Johnson, M. D. Integrative genome analysis reveals an oncomir/oncogene cluster regulating glioblastoma survivorship. Proc Natl Acad Sci U S A. (2010).

[82] Su, B, Cheng, J, Yang, J, & Guo, Z. MEKK2 is required for T-cell receptor signals in JNK activation and interleukin-2 gene expression. J Biol Chem. (2001).

[83] Sasayama, T, Nishihara, M, Kondoh, T, Hosoda, K, & Kohmura, E. MicroRNA-10b is overexpressed in malignant glioma and associated with tumor invasive factors, uPAR and RhoC. Int J Cancer. (2009).

[84] Xia, H, Qi, Y, Ng, S. S, Chen, X, Chen, S, Fang, M, Li, D, Zhao, Y, Ge, R, Li, G, Chen, Y, He, M. L, Kung, H. F, Lai, L, & Lin, M. C. MicroRNA-15b regulates cell cycle progression by targeting cyclins in glioma cells. Biochem Biophys Res Commun. (2009).

[85] Xia, H, Qi, Y, Ng, S. S, Chen, X, Li, D, Chen, S, Ge, R, Jiang, S, Li, G, Chen, Y, He, M. L, Kung, H. F, Lai, L, & Lin, M. C. microRNA-146b inhibits glioma cell migration and invasion by targeting MMPs. Brain Res. (2009).

[86] Würdinger, T, Tannous, BA, Saydam, O, Skog, J, Grau, S, Soutschek, J, Weissleder, R, Breakefield, XO, Krichevsky, AM, & mi, . -296 regulates growth factor receptor overexpression in angiogenic endothelial cells. Cancer Cell. 2008,14(5):382-393.

[87] Navarro, A, Marrades, R. M, Viñolas, N, Quera, A, Agustí, C, Huerta, A, Ramirez, J, Torres, A, & Monzo, M. MicroRNAs expressed during lung cancer development are expressed in human pseudoglandular lung embryogenesis. Oncology. (2009).

[88] Ernst, A, Campos, B, Meier, J, Devens, F, Liesenberg, F, Wolter, M, Reifenberger, G, Herold-mende, C, Lichter, P, & Radlwimmer, B. De-repression of CTGF via the miR-cluster upon differentiation of human glioblastoma spheroid cultures. Oncogene. (2010). , 17-92.

[89] Ferrara, N. Role of vascular endothelial growth factor in physiologic and pathologic angiogenesis: therapeutic implications. Semin Oncol. (2002). Suppl 16):10-14.

[90] Inoki, I, Shiomi, T, Hashimoto, G, Enomoto, H, Nakamura, H, Makino, K, Ikeda, E, Takata, S, Kobayashi, K, & Okada, Y. Connective tissue growth factor binds vascular endothelial growth factor (VEGF) and inhibits VEGF-induced angiogenesis. FASEB J. (2002).

[91] Suárez, Y, Fernández-hernando, C, Yu, J, Gerber, S. A, Harrison, K. D, Pober, J. S, Iruela-arispe, M. L, Merkenschlager, M, & Sessa, W. C. Dicer-dependent endothelial microRNAs are necessary for postnatal angiogenesis. Proc Natl Acad Sci U S A. (2008).

[92] Lee, S. T, Chu, K, Oh, H. J, Im, W. S, Lim, J. Y, Kim, S. K, Park, C. K, Jung, K. H, Lee, S. K, Kim, M, & Roh, J. K. Let-7 microRNA inhibits the proliferation of human glioblastoma cells. J Neurooncol. (2011).

[93] Galli, R, Binda, E, Orfanelli, U, Cipelletti, B, Gritti, A, De Vitis, S, Fiocco, R, Foroni, C, Dimeco, F, & Vescovi, A. Isolation and characterization of tumorigenic, stem-like neural precursors from human glioblastoma. Cancer Res. (2004).

[94] Bao, S, Wu, Q, Mclendon, R. E, Hao, Y, Shi, Q, Hjelmeland, A. B, Dewhirst, M. W, & Bigner, D. D. and Rich JN: Glioma stem cells promote radioresistance by preferential activation of the DNA damage response. Nature.(2006).

[95] Johannessen, T. C, Wang, J, Skaftnesmo, K. O, Sakariassen, P. Ø, Enger, P. Ø, Petersen, K, Øyan, A. M, Kalland, K. H, & Bjerkvig, R. and Tysnes BB: Highly infltrative brain tumours show reduced chemosensitivity associated with a stem cell-like phenotype. Neuropathol Appl Neurobiol.(2009).

[96] Lavon, I, Zrihan, D, Granit, A, Einstein, O, Fainstein, N, Cohen, M. A, Cohen, M. A, Zelikovitch, B, Shoshan, Y, Spektor, S, Reubinoff, B. E, Felig, Y, Gerlitz, O, Ben-hur, T, Smith, Y, & Siegal, T. Gliomas display a microRNA expression profile reminiscent of neural precursor cells. Neurooncology.(2010).

[97] Felsberg, J, Yan, P. S, Huang, T. H, Milde, U, Schramm, J, Wiestler, O. D, Reifenberger, G, Pietsch, T, & Waha, A. DNA methylation and allelic losses on chromosome arm 14q in oligodendroglial tumours. Neuropathol Appl Neurobiol.(2006).

[98] Gal, H, Pandi, G, Kanner, A. A, Ram, Z, Lithwick-yanai, G, Amariglio, N, Rechavi, G, & Givol, D. MIR-451 and Imatinib mesylate inhibit tumor growth of Glioblastoma stem cells. Biochem Biophys Res Commun. (2008).

[99] Hatfield, S. D, Shcherbata, H. R, Fischer, K. A, Nakahara, K, Carthew, R. W, & Ruohola-baker, H. Stem cell division is regulated by the microRNA pathway. Nature. (2005).

[100] Kefas, B, Comeau, L, Erdle, N, Montgomery, E, Amos, S, & Purow, B. Pyruvate kinase M2 is a target of the tumor-suppressive microRNA-326 and regulates the survival of glioma cells. Neuro Oncol. (2010).

[101] Gajjar, A, Hernan, R, Kocak, M, Fuller, C, Lee, Y, Mckinnon, P. J, Wallace, D, Lau, C, Chintagumpala, M, Ashley, D. M, Kellie, S. J, & Kun, L. and Gilbertson RJ: Clinical, histopathologic, and molecular markers of prognosis: toward a new disease risk strati-fcation system for medulloblastoma. J Clin Oncol.(2004).

[102] Johnson, S. M, Grosshans, H, Shingara, J, Byrom, M, Jarvis, R, Cheng, A, Labourier, E, Reinert, K. L, Brown, D, & Slack, F. J. RAS is regulated by the let-7 microRNA family. Cell.(2005).

[103] MacDonald TJBrown KM, LaFleur B, Peterson K, Lawlor C, Chen Y, Packer RJ, Co-gen P, Stephan DA. Expression profiling of medulloblastoma: PDGFRA and the RAS/ MAPK pathway as therapeutic targets for metastatic disease.Nat Genet. (2001).

[104] Ferretti, E, De Smaele, E, & Po, A. Di Marcotullio L, Tosi E, Espinola MS, Di Rocco C, Riccardi R, Giangaspero F, Farcomeni A, Nofroni I, Laneve P, Gioia U, Caffarelli E, Bozzoni I, Screpanti I, Gulino A. MicroRNA profiling in human medulloblastoma. Int J Cancer. (2009).

[105] Visvanathan, J, Lee, S, Lee, B, Lee, J. W, & Lee, S. K. The microRNA miR-124 antago-nizes the anti-neural REST/SCP1 pathway during embryonic CNS development. Genes Dev. (2007).

[106] Lawinger, P, Venugopal, R, Guo, Z. S, Immaneni, A, Sengupta, D, Lu, W, & Rastelli, L. Marin Dias Carneiro A, Levin V, Fuller GN, Echelard Y, Majumder S.The neuronal repressor REST/NRSF is an essential regulator in medulloblastoma cells. Nat Med. (2000).

[107] Fuller, G. N, Su, X, Price, R. E, Cohen, Z. R, Lang, F. F, Sawaya, R, & Majumder, S. Many human medulloblastoma tumors overexpress repressor element-1 silencing transcription (REST)/neuron-restrictive silencer factor, which can be functionally countered by REST-VP16. Mol Cancer Ther. (2005).

[108] Conaco, C, Otto, S, Han, J. J, & Mandel, G. Reciprocal actions of REST and a micro-RNA promote neuronal identity. Proc Natl Acad Sci U S A. (2006).

[109] Mendrzyk, F, Radlwimmer, B, Joos, S, Kokocinski, F, Benner, A, Stange, D. E, Neben, K, Fiegler, H, Carter, N. P, Reifenberger, G, Korshunov, A, & Lichter, P. Genomic and protein expression profiling identifies CDK6 as novel independent prognostic mark-er in medulloblastoma. J Clin Oncol. (2005).

[110] Li, KK, Pang, JC, Ching, AK, Wong, CK, Kong, X, Wang, Y, Zhou, L, Chen, Z, Ng, HK, & mi, . -124 is frequently down-regulated in medulloblastoma and is a negative regulator of SLC16A1. Hum Pathol. 2009,40(9):1234-1243.

[111] Liu, W, Gong, Y. H, Chao, T. F, Peng, X. Z, Yuan, J. G, Ma, Z. Y, Jia, G, & Zhao, J. Z. Identification of differentially expressed microRNAs by microarray: a possible role for microRNAs gene in medulloblastomas. Chin Med J (Engl). (2009).

[112] Ruiz i Altaba ASánchez P, Dahmane N. Gli and hedgehog in cancer: tumours, em-bryos and stem cells. Nat Rev Cancer. (2002).

[113] Kimura, H, Stephen, D, Joyner, A, & Curran, T. Gli1 is important for medulloblasto-ma formation in Ptc1+/- mice. Oncogene. (2005).

[114] Ferretti, E, De Smaele, E, Miele, E, Laneve, P, Po, A, Pelloni, M, & Paganelli, A. Di Marcotullio L, Caffarelli E, Screpanti I, Bozzoni I, Gulino A. Concerted microRNA control of Hedgehog signalling in cerebellar neuronal progenitor and tumour cells. EMBO J. (2008).

[115] Uziel, T, Karginov, F. V, Xie, S, Parker, J. S, Wang, Y. D, Gajjar, A, He, L, Ellison, D, Gilbertson, R. J, Hannon, G, & Roussel, M. F. The miR-17~92 cluster collaborates with the Sonic Hedgehog pathway in medulloblastoma. Proc Natl Acad Sci U S A. (2009).

[116] Northcott, P. A, Fernandez-l, A, Hagan, J. P, Ellison, D. W, Grajkowska, W, Gillespie, Y, Grundy, R, Van Meter, T, Rutka, J. T, Croce, C. M, Kenney, A. M, & Taylor, M. D. The miR-17/92 polycistron is up-regulated in sonic hedgehog-driven medulloblastomas and induced by N-myc in sonic hedgehog-treated cerebellar neural precursors. Cancer Res. (2009).

[117] Solecki, D. J, Liu, X. L, Tomoda, T, Fang, Y, & Hatten, M. E. Activated Notch2 signaling inhibits differentiation of cerebellar granule neuron precursors by maintaining proliferation. Neuron. (2001).

[118] Ishibashi, M, Moriyoshi, K, Sasai, Y, Shiota, K, Nakanishi, S, & Kageyama, R. Persistent expression of helix-loop-helix factor HES-1 prevents mammalian neural differentiation in the central nervous system. EMBO J. (1994).

[119] Garzia, L, Andolfo, I, Cusanelli, E, Marino, N, Petrosino, G, De Martino, D, Esposito, V, Galeone, A, Navas, L, Esposito, S, Gargiulo, S, Fattet, S, Donofrio, V, Cinalli, G, Brunetti, A, Vecchio, L. D, Northcott, P. A, Delattre, O, Taylor, M. D, Iolascon, A, & Zollo, M. MicroRNA-199b-5p impairs cancer stem cells through negative regulation of HES1 in medulloblastoma. PLoS One. (2009). e4998.

[120] Venkataraman, S, Alimova, I, Fan, R, Harris, P, Foreman, N, & Vibhakar, R. MicroRNA 128a increases intracellular ROS level by targeting Bmi-1 and inhibits medulloblastoma cancer cell growth by promoting senescence. PLoS One. (2010). e10748.

[121] Diehn, M, Cho, R. W, Lobo, N. A, Kalisky, T, Dorie, M. J, Kulp, A. N, Qian, D, Lam, J. S, Ailles, L. E, Wong, M, Joshua, B, Kaplan, M. J, Wapnir, I, Dirbas, F. M, Somlo, G, Garberoglio, C, Paz, B, Shen, J, Lau, S. K, Quake, S. R, Brown, J. M, Weissman, I. L, & Clarke, M. F. Association of reactive oxygen species levels and radioresistance in cancer stem cells. Nature. (2009).

[122] Vandeva, S, Jaffrain-rea, M. L, Daly, A. F, Tichomirowa, M, Zacharieva, S, & Beckers, A. The genetics of pituitary adenomas. Best Pract Res Clin Endocrinol Metab. (2010).

[123] Bottoni, A, Piccin, D, Tagliati, F, Luchin, A, & Zatelli, M. C. degli Uberti EC. miR-15a and miR-down-regulation in pituitary adenomas. J Cell Physiol. (2005). , 16-1.

[124] Fan, X, Paetau, A, Aalto, Y, Välimäki, M, Sane, T, Poranen, A, Castresana, J. S, & Knuutila, S. Gain of chromosome 3 and loss of 13q are frequent alterations in pituitary adenomas. Cancer Genet Cytogenet. (2001).

[125] Cimmino, A, Calin, GA, Fabbri, M, Iorio, MV, Ferracin, M, Shimizu, M, Wojcik, SE, Aqeilan, RI, Zupo, S, Dono, M, Rassenti, L, Alder, H, Volinia, S, Liu, CG, Kipps, TJ, Negrini, M, Croce, CM, & mi, . -16 induce apoptosis by targeting BCL2. Proc Natl Acad Sci U S A. 2005,102(39):13944-13949.

[126] Wang, D. G, Johnston, C. F, Atkinson, A. B, Heaney, A. P, Mirakhur, M, & Buchanan, K. D. Expression of bcl-2 oncoprotein in pituitary tumours: comparison with c-myc. J Clin Pathol. (1996).

[127] Bottoni, A, Zatelli, M. C, Ferracin, M, Tagliati, F, Piccin, D, Vignali, C, Calin, G. A, Negrini, M, & Croce, C. M. Degli Uberti EC. Identification of differentially expressed microRNAs by microarray: a possible role for microRNA genes in pituitary adenomas. J Cell Physiol. (2007).

[128] Amaral, F. C, Torres, N, Saggioro, F, Neder, L, & Machado, H. R. Silva WA Jr, Moreira AC, Castro M. MicroRNAs differentially expressed in ACTH-secreting pituitary tumors. J Clin Endocrinol Metab. (2009).

[129] Zhou, G, Bao, Z. Q, & Dixon, J. E. Components of a new human protein kinase signal transduction pathway. J Biol Chem. (1995).

[130] Qian, Z. R, Asa, S. L, Siomi, H, Siomi, M. C, Yoshimoto, K, Yamada, S, Wang, E. L, Rahman, M. M, Inoue, H, Itakura, M, Kudo, E, & Sano, T. Overexpression of HMGA2 relates to reduction of the let-7 and its relationship to clinicopathological features in pituitary adenomas. Mod Pathol. (2009).

[131] Lee, Y. S, & Dutta, A. The tumor suppressor microRNA let-7 represses the HMGA2 oncogene. Genes Dev. (2007).

[132] Pierantoni, G. M, Finelli, P, Valtorta, E, Giardino, D, Rodeschini, O, Esposito, F, Losa, M, Fusco, A, & Larizza, L. High-mobility group A2 gene expression is frequently induced in non-functioning pituitary adenomas (NFPAs), even in the absence of chromosome 12 polysomy. Endocr Relat Cancer. (2005).

[133] Butz, H, Likó, I, Czirják, S, Igaz, P, Khan, M. M, Zivkovic, V, Bálint, K, Korbonits, M, Rácz, K, & Patócs, A. Down-regulation of Wee1 kinase by a specific subset of microRNA in human sporadic pituitary adenomas. J Clin Endocrinol Metab. (2010). E, 181-91.

[134] Stenvang, J, Petri, A, Lindow, M, Obad, S, & Kauppinen, S. Inhibition of microRNA function by antimiR oligonucleotides. Silence. (2012).

[135] Ebert, M. S, Neilson, J. R, & Sharp, P. A. MicroRNA sponges: competitive inhibitors of small RNAs in mammalian cells. Nat Methods. (2007).

[136] Lennox, K. A, & Behlke, M. A. Chemical modification and design of anti-miRNA oligonucleotides. Gene Ther. (2011).

[137] Esau, C. C. Inhibition of microRNA with antisense oligonucleotides. Methods. (2008).

[138] Corsten, M. F, Miranda, R, Kasmieh, R, Krichevsky, A. M, Weissleder, R, & Shah, K. MicroRNA-21 knockdown disrupts glioma growth in vivo and displays synergistic cytotoxicity with neural precursor cell delivered S-TRAIL in human gliomas. Cancer Res. (2007).

[139] Würdinger, T, Tannous, BA, Saydam, O, Skog, J, Grau, S, Soutschek, J, Weissleder, R, Breakefield, XO, Krichevsky, AM, & mi, . -296 regulates growth factor receptor over-expression in angiogenic endothelial cells. Cancer Cell. 2008,14(5):382-393.

Chapter 4

Evolvement of microRNAs as Therapeutic Targets for Malignant Gliomas

Sihan Wu, Wenbo Zhu and Guangmei Yan

Additional information is available at the end of the chapter

1. Introduction

Malignant glioma (MG), consisting of anaplastic glioma (AA, WHO grade III) and glioblastomamultiforme (GBM, WHO grade IV, 60-70%), is the most common and destructive brain tumor [1]. Despite systemic treatment, surgical resection followed by radiotherapy and chemotherapy, the prognosis of patients with GBM remains poor with a median survival of 12 to 15 months and a 5-year survival rate of 9.8% [2, 3]. The dismal outcome fuels the need to understand the molecular basis of gliomagenesis and identify novel therapeutic targets for MG treatment.

With a developing understanding of core aberrant signaling pathways in MG, molecular targeted therapy has shown certain promise as a more rational strategy. Established targets, including receptor tyrosine kinases (RTK) such as EGFR, PDGFR and VEGFR, as well as mTOR, farnesyl transferase and PI3K, have drawn particular interests both in fundamental and clinical research. However, single targeted agents so far have not displayed desirable clinical outcomes as expected, with response rates of 0 to 15% and no prolongation of 6-month progression-free survival [4–6]. This disappointing outcome is primarily due to the nature of cancer with multi-genetic abnormality and inter/intra-tumor heterogeneity. Therefore, multiple targeting strategies are essential to achieve better clinical benefits.

MicroRNA (miRNA), a type of endogenous small non-coding RNA which negatively modulates gene expression in post-transcriptional level, has rapidly become a topical issue since it was firstly discovered in *C. elegans* two decades ago[7]. Increasing researches have reported that dysregulation of miRNA is closely associated with tumorigenesis and tumor progression. In gliomas, a group of miRNAs have been characterized as oncogenic and tumor-suppressive molecules. With a unique feature of multi-targeting, miRNA may become a new powerful weapon fighting against MG. Although much remains to be learned about formulating miRNAs as nucleic acid drugs, we feel that identification of miRNAs as therapeutic targets for gliomas is now within sight.

In this chapter, we will critically review issues relevant to contemporary researches on miR-NAs and MG. Based upon other teams' and our data, this review will present findings on oncogenic and tumor-suppressive properties of miRNA in MG, focusing on the mechanisms of dysregulation, the involvement with core pathways of MG and the functional heterogeneity in different context. Besides, we will formulate evidences for miRNA-based clinical application in diagnosis and therapeutics of MG. The developing cognition of miRNAs will ultimately lead to innovative clinical approaches for MG.

2. Oncogenic and tumor-suppressive miRNAs in malignant gliomas

The very first oncogenic miRNA indentified in GBM is miR-21 as early as 2005 [8], although whose target genes were not fully understood at that time. In 2008, another group identified a set of targets of this miRNA which constitute a tumor-suppressive network including TGF-β, p53 and mitochondrial-apoptotic pathways [9]. This is one of the examples showing the multi-targeting nature of miRNAs in oncology. Beyond multi-targeting, these findings also prompt a hypothesis that miRNAs may have pathway preference in some cases.

Coincidently, also in 2005, S.A. Ciafre*et al.* firstly described that brain-enriched miR-128 and miR-181 family were frequently down-regulated in primary GBMs and cell lines [10], whose tumor-suppressive roles of these miRNAs were subsequently validated in the next few years [11–14].

In 2008, a milestone has been made in glioma research, accomplished by The Cancer Genome Atlas (TCGA) Research Network. Through integrative analysis of DNA copy number, gene expression and DNA methylation aberrations, TCGA defined three major pathways in GBM, which are RTK, p53 and RB signaling pathways, as shown in Figure 1 [15]. These pathways cannot be more familiar to every oncologist: frequently activated RTK signaling in cancer supports cell proliferation and survival, whereas p53 and RB signaling monitor cell cycle transition and couple to apoptosis and senescence pathways, which are commonly suppressed in cancer. To date, increasing oncogenic and tumor-suppressive miRNAs in MGs have been uncovered. In combination with genomic sketch of GBM described by TCGA, we have a deeper insight into the interactions within the core pathways of MG, which are controlled in coding and non-coding levels (Figure 1).

Here we do not pay our attention to the detail of each single miRNA, since several reviews have provided considerable details about their expression and function [16–18]. In this paper, we prefer to focus on how these miRNAs become aberrant, and which malignant phenotypes they contribute to.

As well as every protein coding gene, non-coding miRNA genes may similarly undergo over or lost expression, amplification, deletion, insertion, translocation and mutation, which lead to aberration of miRNAs. The mechanisms of miRNA aberration have not yet been extensively studied. Nevertheless, there have been some clues showing that transcriptional activity, single nucleotide polymorphism (SNP) and chromosome deletion contribute to aberrant genotype and malignant phenotype of MG.

The most interesting research addressing miRNA transcriptional regulation machinery in MGs is the *TP53* and miR-25/32 feedback circuitry [19]. Carlo M. Croce's and co-workers found that miR-25 and miR-32 are negatively regulated by *TP53* via repressing their transcriptional factors *MYC* and *E2F1*. Intriguingly, by directly targeting *MDM2* and *TSC1*, these miRNAs help stabilize P53 protein and suppress tumorigenicity in U87 GBM cells. Thus, a fine tuned recurrent autoregulatory circuit form. However, in the non-functional mutant *TP53* context, miR-25/32 support cell proliferation *per contra*. These findings not only provide insights into the interaction between miRNAs and *TP53* tumor-suppressive pathway, but also hint that a given miRNA may have distinct function in different genetic and biochemical status.

It is unexpected that miRNA genes rarely exhibit SNP or mutation within the major mature sequence segment, although which can be commonly found in the precursor (including the minor mature sequence which is formerly called the star sequence) and primary miRNA segments. Through mining human SNP database, Peng Jin's group identified a G>U polymorphism located in the eighth nucleotide of the mature miR-125a-5p. The U allele blocks the processing from pri-miRNA to miRNA precursor by altering the secondary structure, and impairs miRNA-mediated translational suppression [20]. MiR-125s have been demonstrated to be tumor-suppressive in GBM [21–23]. However, such nucleotide alteration has not yet been described in glioma clinical data. The rs11614913 SNP, which locates in the segment producing minor mature miR-196a-3p (termed miR-196a* previously), was firstly found to be associated with the risk of glioma in Chinese population [24]. Recent clinical study indicates that the rs2910164 in segment containing minor mature miR-146a-3p sequence is also relative to the risk and prognosis in adult glioma [25]. These findings improve our understandings of miRNA-related pathogenesis and diagnostics in gliomas. Further research is required to fully comprehend the exact mechanisms underlying the relationship between miRNA gene SNPs and clinical outcomes, which may have huge clinical potential.

Chromosome alteration undoubtedly contributes to miRNA aberration. Particularly in diffuse astrocytoma (DA, WHO II) and AA, chromosome 7q32 is a hotspot that frequently amplifies. This region embraces eight miRNAs: miR-593, miR-129-1, miR-335, miR-182, miR-96, miR-183, miR-29a and miR-29b-1. Among these miRNAs, our group recently reported that miR-335 is the most striking target in AA [26]. We have demonstrated that miR-335 confers invasive and proliferative malignant phenotype on astrocytoma via targeting *DAAM1*. Disrupting miR-335 by cholesterylated miRNA inhibitor abrogates invasion and elicits apoptosis both *in vitro* and *in vivo*. Chromosome amplification in cancer often creates abnormal high level of coding and non-coding products that subsequently infests the well-balanced signaling. Currently, drug screening and discovery in oncology specifically focus on overexpressed protein and over-activated kinase. We believe that miRNA, such as miR-335, may also be the target for drug development in the future.

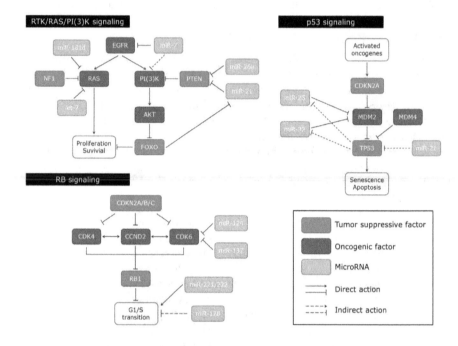

Figure 1. Interaction between microRNAs and core pathways in malignant gliomas.

3. Dual scripts for a miRNA

In the last session we have mentioned that miR-25/32 functions differently depended on *TP53* status in GBM. It is not the sole evidence that a given miRNA plays distinct roles in respective models. In fact, miRNAs show complicated functional heterogeneity.

One of the examples is miR-135a/b. Remco Nagel *et al.* found increased expression levels of miR-135a and miR-135b during colorectal cancer progression, which target the tumor suppressor gene Adenomatous Polyposis Coli (*APC*)[27]. The oncogenic role of miR-135a was further confirmed by BR Zetter's group. They demonstrated that paclitaxel resistance is associated with up-regulation of miR-135a in multiple solid tumor cell lines. Knocking-down of miR-135a acquires susceptibility to paclitaxel[28]. However, in classic Hodgkin lymphoma (cHL), miR-135a directly regulates *JAK2*, thus suppressing the expression of *BCL2L1* (also known as *BCL-XL*) and inducing apoptosis. Furthermore, higher level of miR-135a indicates better disease-free survival in cHL patients [29]. Likewise our group has also characterized that miR-135a functions as a selective killer of MG. We have reported that glial cell-enriched miR-135a is frequently down-regulated in MG and negatively correlates with the pathological grading of gliomas. Ectopic delivery of miR-135a selectively triggers mito-chondrial dependent apoptosis in MG *in vitro* and *in vivo*. Interestingly, this lethal effect is neutral in normal glial cells and neurons [30].

MiR-335 gives us another example of the dual role nature of miRNAs. An early study identi-fied that miR-335 suppresses breast cancer metastasis and migration through targeting *SOX4* and *TNC* [31]. However, as mentioned above, our recent research found that this miR-NA promotes invasion and proliferation in AA [26]. In this way, miRNAs seems to have cell-type-dependent functional heterogeneity. The definition of "tumor-suppressive" and "oncogenic" should be carefully employed depended on the cell types and diseases.

Even within the same cell type, the functional behavior of a given miRNA can also be di-verse. Previously we have reported that activation of cAMP/PKA pathway, manipulated by Cholera toxin, induces cellular differentiation of MG, showing malignant phenotype rever-sion and potent GFAP (glial fibrillary acidic protein) expression [32]. As it has been well characterized, we found that IL-6/JAK2/STAT3 contributes to GFAP expression in this mod-el [33]. Notably, epigenetic mechanism is also involved. In this context, the so-called onco-genic miR-335 in MG induced by Cholera toxin enhances GFAP expression in MG cell lines and primary cultures [34]. Multi-targeting is one of the natures of miRNAs. Signaling net-works composed of target genes and their relative molecules may both contribute to tumor-suppressive and oncogenic function. It seems that the oncogenic functions of miR-335 are hindered under a high endogenous level of cAMP, rewiring to pro-differentiation pathways.

To sum up, the role of a given miRNA depends on the script which is assigned by the cell type, the genomic context and in part the cellular biochemical status. These observations re-mind that disease state as well as the genomic subclass of MGs should be considered in the preclinical study especially for drug discovery involved miRNAs.

4. Involvement of miRNAs as novel biomarkers in malignant gliomas

Biomarkers are distinctive biological indicators that serve for diagnosis, prognosis and med-ication. Traditional biomarkers include mRNAs, proteins and metabolites. At present, miR-NAs are emerging as novel and practical biomarkers in oncology. Due to their surprising stability, miRNAs can not only be detected in fresh and frozen tissues, but also in body flu-ids and even formalin-fixed paraffin-embedded samples. In the study of Roland Schroers, miR-15b and miR-21 are found in cerebrospinal fluid and demonstrated to be markers of glioma [35]. Although much remains to be studied, *e.g.* to discover more accurate and specif-ic markers for respective glioma types, this finding provides a new opportunity to develop less invasive and early diagnostic approach for gliomas.

Besides diagnosis, miRNAs may be promising biomarkers for prognosis. Jun Li's group has reported that miR-182 is markedly up-regulated in various glioma cell lines and primary glioma specimens. Furthermore, higher level of miR-182 is associated with poor overall sur-vival of patients with malignant glioma [36]. A more comprehensive study was recently carried out by Sujaya Srinivasan, *et al*. They analyzed miRNA expression profile of GBM patients (n = 222) from TCGA database and found a ten-miRNA expression signature that predicts survival for GBM. In detail, three miRNAs (miR-20a, miR-106a and miR-17-5p) were identified as protective markers and seven miRNAs (hsa-miR-31, hsa-miR-222, hsa-miR-148a, hsa-miR-221, hsa-miR-146b, hsa-miR-200b and hsa-miR-193a) were risky [37].

Recent studies have raised a possibility that miRNAs may function as predictive markers for therapeutics. Temozolomide (TMZ) is a well-known alkylating agent against gliomas, which methylates guanines in the O-6 position. Accumulating O-6 methyl guanines lead to DNA mismatch during replication and ultimately result in cell death. Although *MGMT* (methyl-guanine methyl transferase) promoter methylation has been proved to be a strongest marker to predict the TMZ response in low-grade and high-grade gliomas [38–40], it may not be the only indicator. Recent research indicates that miR-181b/c, miR-195, miR-455-3p and miR-10a-3p, rather than MGMT promoter methylation, predict response to concomitant che-moradiotherapy and acquired TMZ resistance in GBM cell line and patients [41, 42]. In addition, increasing evidences indicate that miRNAs also contribute to other drug response. For instance, up-regulated miR-21 confers teniposide and paclitaxel resistance on GBM cells [43, 44]. Various highly efficient MGMT inhibitors have been developed for sensitizing tumor to TMZ [45]. The emerging roles of miRNAs in drug resistance of TMZ and other antineoplastic agents give us a novel angle to include miRNAs as therapeutic targets.

5. Perspectives on miRNAs as nucleic acid drugs in malignant gliomas

5.1. MiRNAs replacement therapy and suppressive therapy

Human body has an extremely complicated internal environment, relying on balance and stability of which human keep their health. Once the homeostasis is disrupted by down-regulation or up-regulation of some important molecules including miRNAs, human will suffer from all kinds of diseases. Based on the disequilibrium status, the ideal protocols to cure diseases are believed to replace what is lost and to repress what is excessive, which are respectively called replacement therapy and suppressive therapy. For the former, estrogen replacement therapy is the most representative example, which is generally used in menopausal women with menopausal syndrome caused by ovarian hormones loss and has shown a positive effect [46]. For the latter, a typical case is a famous anti-angiogenesis drug Avastin, the humanized anti-vascular endothelial growth factor (VEGF) monoclonal antibody for cancer therapy [47]. Besides, Gefitinib and Glivec specially inhibiting EGFR tyrosine kinase, have both achieved high clinical benefit rates in treating cancer especially lung carcinoma and chronic myelocytic leukemia[48,49], further indicating the efficacy of suppressive therapy via targeting core molecules in tumorigenesis.

Notably, increasing evidences demonstrated that gliomagenesis is also closely associated with deregulation of miRNAs, such as up-regulation of oncogenic miRNAs and down-regulation of tumor suppressive miRNAs. Therefore, targeting these aberrant miRNAs has tremendous potential as a therapeutic strategy by down- or up-regulating altered genes.

Specially, miRNA mimics can be synthesized to replace lessened ones critical in gliomagenesis, and miRNA inhibitors can be designed to suppress the function of up-regulated oncogenic miRNAs. Just less than two decades after discovering the role of miRNAs in oncology, the replacement and suppressive therapies of miRNA are already being used in preclinical researches. We have proved that artificially rectification of abnormally expressed miRNAs inhibited growth of glioma xenografts in mice and prolonged the median survival of rat with orthotopic glioma[26,30], opening a new sight for glioma treatment.

5.2. MiRNA-targeting cocktail therapy

Glioma is a complicated disease of altered genes. TCGA has reported multiple chromosomal aberrations, nucleotide substitutions and epigenetic modifications that construct three core pathways (as shown in Figure 1] [15]. Furthermore, glioma is a disease of altered miRNAs. A genome-wide expression profiling of 26 GBMs, 13 AAs and 7 normal brain samples identifies multiple deregulated miRNAs in MGs [50]. In addition, large scale of sequencing analysis of GBMs has identified extensive genetic heterogeneity between GBM samples from different patients [51], implying the possibility of miRNA's heterogeneity. The multiplicity of deregulated miRNAs and the heterogeneity of deregulated miRNAs expression profiling may foster therapeutic failure and tumor adaptation to solo miRNA-targeting therapy.

To date, researchers just verified the efficiency of targeting solo miRNA as if by prior agreement. What will happen if target several pivotal miRNAs simultaneously? Given the multiplicity of deregulated miRNAs in glioma, a cocktail consisting of special miRNA mimics and/or inhibitors may kill multiple birds with one stone. In another word, components in cocktail may have an additive effect or even a synergistic effect against MGs. Furthermore, considering individual differences, one cocktail may not fit for each patient with MGs. If we can design a specific miRNA cocktail based on individual deregulated miRNAs, miRNA individualized treatment will be within our sights. Certainly, additional preliminary evidences are needed to verify the feasibility and availability of miRNA-targeting cocktail therapeutics.

5.3. Engineering miRNA

Engineering miRNA (emiRNA) is artificially designed in sequence, endowed with functional similarity to natural miRNA and functional specificity according to human's will. In a sense, emiRNA is a branch of small interfering RNA (siRNA) that possesses multi-targeting power just as natural miRNA.

Leastwise, there are two strategies to design emiRNA: (a) adjustment based on the natural miRNA sequence; (b) *de novo* design.

In the sessions above, we have discussed the fact that a given miRNA may play distinct role in different models, *e.g.* different genetic background, different cell type and different second messenger level. Even in a "conclusive"circumstance that a certain miRNA strongly kills a type of cancer cell, we still need to evaluate its pharmacodynamics in the cancer tissue and toxic side effect to the normal tissue before clinical application. If a natural sequence miRNA shows remarkable antitumor effect but exhibits unsatisfying selectivity, does it mean we should totally abandon this target? The problem may be solved by emiRNA technology. Different dominant target genes and their roles in different models determine the functional heterogeneity of a given miRNA. If we are able to find out the undesired targets that lead to unsatisfying selectivity, perhaps by keeping the seed region of the miRNA and adjusting its 3' nucleotide sequence, we could either avoid the interaction between the miRNA and the undesired target genes, or enhance the binding to our goal targets.

In broader context, we could design an artificial miRNA in a *de nove* way. Cancers are known as a type of multigenic disease. By comprehensive sequencing, RTK/RAS/PI[3]K, p53 and RBsignalings are characterized as the core pathways in GBM [15]. In virtue of bioinformatics, it is possible to design a miRNA that contemporaneously targets the key components of two or more pathways by carefully examining their mutual microRNA recognition elements (MREs).

However, numbers of scientific problems need to be addressed before putting emiRNA into practice. We still have limited knowledge about the details of miRNA biogenesis and the MRE language passing on along evolution. Someday the secret will be unlocked and emiRNA may be a practical weapon against cancers.

5.4. MiRNA formulation

Another attractive issue of translating miRNA into clinical application is formulation. Although whose length is quite short in the RNA world, miRNA as well as siRNA is a type of high molecular weight drug in pharmaceutical point of view. Additionally, electric charge contributed by phosphate groups of the nucleic acid backbone make it inadequate for CNS delivery. Fortunately, new technical progress brings miRNA formulation within sight.

In the earlier period, viral vector including retrovirus, adenovirus, herpes simplex virus and adeno-associated virus were broadly used due to their high efficiency for both gene delivery and expression. However, limitations associated with safety, genomic stability and immunogenicity motivate scientists to focus on non-viral systems. At present, remarkable achievements have been made in chemical modifications and conjugations of small RNA. For example, locked nucleic acid (LNA) technology not only increases melting temperature of RNA-RNA duplex thus enhancing the binding affinity between small RNA and target transcript, but also improves the half-life of small RNA in serum, which is critical for therapeutic use [52]. Cholesterylation, *viz.* modification with cholesteryl functionality, which improves the cellular uptake of small RNA, is now extensively used for miRNA mimics/inhibitors and siRNA in preclinical research [53]. Two reviews have provided clear and comprehensive introduction of the progress on chemical small RNA encapsulation [54, 55]. Particularly, a recent study from Paula Hammond and colleagues reported a self-assembled microsponges of small RNA hairpin polymersin corporated more than half a million copies of siRNA in a single nanoparticle [56]. This novel technology allow one thousand times lower concentration to achieve same degree of gene silencing efficiency as conventional strategies, showing great clinical application potential. In the near future, small RNA formulation will further benefit from evolution of nanotechnology and biomaterial technology.

6. Concluding remark

Glioma is not the type of high incidence disease; however the depressive clinical outcomes still threaten human health. Special location, rapid proliferation, invasive growth and massive angiogenesis are the key issues that limit treatment for MG. In addition, extremely complicated histopathological and genomic classifications perplex fundamental and clinical research.

With the evolution of new generation high through-put sequencing technology, clearer insights of driver mutations and core pathways in various cancers are gradually revealed in the recent period [57–59]. According to these cancer genomic studies, we realize that not only aberrant coding genes lead to cancers, but also non-coding components underneath the iceberg. Twenty-year's research on miRNA opens a new world of genetics and oncology. More and more groups are dedicated to study the role of miRNA in cancer including glioma. Albeit fragmentary, accumulating data will offer deeper insights of glioma with more systematic considerations.

Compared with other non-coding protagonists, *e.g.* histone modification and DNA methylation, miRNA is the easiest role to be specifically manipulated, either by over-expression or inhibition, which determines miRNA to be the star with enormous clinical potential. Although we have not drawn an elaborate picture of miRNA biogenesis, especially how primary sequence and intra-cellular microenvironment influence secondary structure and eventually contribute to processing and maturation, as well as the communication principles between miRNA and MRE, we believe that technologies nowadays are poised to uncover the law of miRNA in oncology. We envision that this intrinsic biomolecule will be the therapeutic target for cancer.

Author details

Sihan Wu, Wenbo Zhu and Guangmei Yan

Zhongshan School of Medicine, Sun Yat-sen University, People's Republic of China

References

[1] Louis, D.N., Ohgaki, H., Wiestler, O.D., Cavenee WK. WHO Classification of Tumours of the Central Nervous System. IARC Press; 2007.

[2] Meyer M a. Malignant Gliomas in Adults. New England Journal of Medicine. 2008 Oct 23;359(17):1850–1850.

[3]   Wirth T, Samaranayake H, Pikkarainen J, Määttä A-M, Ylä-Herttuala S. Clinical trials for glioblastomamultiforme using adenoviral vectors. Current opinion in molecular therapeutics. 2009 Oct;11(5):485–92.

[4]   Sathornsumetee S, Rich JN, Reardon DA. Diagnosis and treatment of high-grade astrocytoma. Neurologic clinics. 2007 Nov;25(4):1111–39, x.

[5]   Chi AS, Wen PY. Inhibiting kinases in malignant gliomas. Expert opinion on therapeutic targets. 2007 Apr;11(4):473–96.

[6]   Sathornsumetee S, Reardon DA, Desjardins A, Quinn JA, Vredenburgh JJ, Rich JN. Molecularly targeted therapy for malignant glioma. Cancer. 2007 Jul 1;110(1):13–24.

[7]   Lee RC, Feinbaum RL, Ambros V. The C. elegansheterochronic gene lin-4 encodes small RNAs with antisense complementarity to lin-14. Cell. 1993 Dec;75(5):843–54.

[8]   Chan J a, Krichevsky AM, Kosik KS. MicroRNA-21 is an antiapoptotic factor in human glioblastoma cells. Cancer research. 2005 Jul 15;65(14):6029–33.

[9]   Papagiannakopoulos T, Shapiro A, Kosik KS. MicroRNA-21 targets a network of key tumor-suppressive pathways in glioblastoma cells. Cancer research. 2008 Oct 1;68(19):8164–72.

[10] Ciafrè SA, Galardi S, Mangiola a, Ferracin M, Liu C-G, Sabatino G, et al. Extensive modulation of a set of microRNAs in primary glioblastoma. Biochemical and biophysical research communications. 2005 Sep 9;334(4):1351–8.

[11] Godlewski J, Nowicki MO, Bronisz A, Williams S, Otsuki A, Nuovo G, et al. Targeting of the Bmi-1 oncogene/stem cell renewal factor by microRNA-128 inhibits glioma proliferation and self-renewal. Cancer research. 2008 Nov 15;68(22):9125–30.

[12] Zhang Y, Chao T, Li R, Liu W, Chen Y, Yan X, et al. MicroRNA-128 inhibits glioma cells proliferation by targeting transcription factor E2F3a. Journal of molecular medicine (Berlin, Germany). 2009 Jan;87(1):43–51.

[13] Shi L, Cheng Z, Zhang J, Li R, Zhao P, Fu Z, et al. hsa-mir-181a and hsa-mir-181b function as tumor suppressors in human glioma cells. Brain research. 2008 Oct 21;1236:185–93.

[14] Wang X-F, Shi Z-M, Wang X-R, Cao L, Wang Y-Y, Zhang J-X, et al. MiR-181d acts as a tumor suppressor in glioma by targeting K-ras and Bcl-2. Journal of cancer research and clinical oncology. 2012 Apr;138(4):573–84.

[15] Cancer T, Atlas G, Information S. Comprehensive genomic characterization defines human glioblastoma genes and core pathways. Nature. 2008 Oct 23;455(7216):1061–8.

[16] Zhang Y, Dutta A. The role of microRNAs in glioma initiation and progression. Frontiers in Bioscience. 2012;700–12.

[17] Pang JC, Kwok WK, Chen Z, Ng H-K. Oncogenic role of microRNAs in brain tumors. Actaneuropathologica. 2009 Jul;117(6):599–611.

[18] Silber J, James CD, Hodgson JG. microRNAs in gliomas: small regulators of a big problem. Neuromolecular medicine. 2009 Jan;11(3):208–22.

[19] Suh S-S, Yoo JY, Nuovo GJ, Jeon Y-J, Kim S, Lee TJ, et al. MicroRNAs/TP53 feedback circuitry in glioblastomamultiforme. Proceedings of the National Academy of Sciences of the United States of America. 2012 Apr 3;109(14):5316–21.

[20] Duan R, Pak C, Jin P. Single nucleotide polymorphism associated with mature miR-125a alters the processing of pri-miRNA. Human molecular genetics. 2007 May 1;16(9):1124–31.

[21] Xia H, He T, Liu C, Cui Y, Song P, Jin X, et al. Cellular Physiology Biochemistry and Biochemistr y MiR-125b Expression Affects the Proliferation and Apoptosis of Human Glioma Cells by Targeting Bmf. Cellular Physiology and Biochemistry. 2009;100081:347–58.

[22] Shi L, Zhang J, Pan T, Zhou J, Gong W, Liu N, et al. MiR-125b is critical for the suppression of human U251 glioma stem cell proliferation. Brain research. Elsevier B.V.; 2010 Feb 2;1312:120–6.

[23] Cortez MA, Nicoloso MS, Shimizu M, Rossi S, Gopisetty G, Molina JR, et al. miR-29b and miR-125a regulate podoplanin and suppress invasion in glioblastoma. Genes, chromosomes & cancer. 2010 Nov;49(11):981–90.

[24] Dou T, Wu Q, Chen X, Ribas J, Ni X, Tang C, et al. A polymorphism of microRNA196a genome region was associated with decreased risk of glioma in Chinese population. Journal of cancer research and clinical oncology. 2010 Dec;136(12):1853–9.

[25] Permuth-Wey J, Thompson RC, Burton Nabors L, Olson JJ, Browning JE, Madden MH, et al. A functional polymorphism in the pre-miR-146a gene is associated with risk and prognosis in adult glioma. Journal of neuro-oncology. 2011 Dec;105(3):639–46.

[26] Shu M, Zheng X, Wu S, Lu H, Leng T, Zhu W, et al. Targeting oncogenic miR-335 inhibits growth and invasion of malignant astrocytoma cells. Molecular cancer. BioMed Central Ltd; 2011 Jan;10(1):59.

[27] Nagel R, le Sage C, Diosdado B, van der Waal M, Oude Vrielink J a F, Bolijn A, et al. Regulation of the adenomatous polyposis coli gene by the miR-135 family in colorectal cancer. Cancer research. 2008 Jul 15;68(14):5795–802.

[28] Holleman a, Chung I, Olsen RR, Kwak B, Mizokami a, Saijo N, et al. miR-135a contributes to paclitaxel resistance in tumor cells both in vitro and in vivo. Oncogene. Nature Publishing Group; 2011 May 9;(September 2010):1–13.

[29] Navarro A, Diaz T, Martinez A, Gaya A, Pons A, Gel B, et al. Regulation of JAK2 by miR-135a: prognostic impact in classic Hodgkin lymphoma. Blood. 2009 Oct 1;114(14):2945–51.

[30] Wu S, Lin Y, Xu D, Chen J, Shu M, Zhou Y, et al. MiR-135a functions as a selective killer of malignant glioma. Oncogene. 2011 Dec 5;31(34):3866–74.

[31] Tavazoie SF, Alarcón C, Oskarsson T, Padua D, Wang Q, Bos PD, et al. Endogenous human microRNAs that suppress breast cancer metastasis. Nature. 2008 Jan 10;451(7175):147–52.

[32] Li Y, Yin W, Wang X, Zhu W, Huang Y, Yan G. Cholera toxin induces malignant glioma cell differentiation via the PKA/CREB pathway. Proceedings of the National Academy of Sciences of the United States of America. 2007 Aug 14;104(33):13438–43.

[33] Shu M, Zhou Y, Zhu W, Wu S, Zheng X, Yan G. Activation of a pro-survival pathway IL-6/JAK2/STAT3 contributes to glial fibrillary acidic protein induction during the cholera toxin-induced differentiation of C6 malignant glioma cells. Molecular oncology. Elsevier B.V; 2011 Jun;5(3):265–72.

[34] Shu M, Zhou Y, Zhu W, Zhang H, Wu S, Chen J, et al. MicroRNA 335 is required for differentiation of malignant glioma cells induced by activation of cAMP/protein kinase A pathway. Molecular pharmacology. 2012 Mar;81(3):292–8.

[35] Baraniskin A, Kuhnhenn J, Schlegel U, Maghnouj A, Zöllner H, Schmiegel W, et al. Identification of microRNAs in the cerebrospinal fluid as biomarker for the diagnosis of glioma. Neuro-oncology. 2012 Jan;14(1):29–33.

[36] Jiang L, Mao P, Song L, Wu J, Huang J, Lin C, et al. miR-182 as a prognostic marker for glioma progression and patient survival. The American journal of pathology. 2010 Jul;177(1):29–38.

[37] Srinivasan S, Patric IRP, Somasundaram K. A ten-microRNA expression signature predicts survival in glioblastoma. PloS one. 2011 Jan;6(3):e17438.

[38] Everhard S, Kaloshi G, Crinière E, Benouaich-Amiel A, Lejeune J, Marie Y, et al. MGMT methylation: a marker of response to temozolomide in low-grade gliomas. Annals of neurology. 2006 Dec;60(6):740–3.

[39] Hegi ME, Diserens A-C, Gorlia T, Hamou M-F, de Tribolet N, Weller M, et al. MGMT gene silencing and benefit from temozolomide in glioblastoma. The New England journal of medicine. 2005 Mar 10;352(10):997–1003.

[40] Stupp R, Hegi ME, Mason WP, van den Bent MJ, Taphoorn MJB, Janzer RC, et al. Effects of radiotherapy with concomitant and adjuvant temozolomide versus radiotherapy alone on survival in glioblastoma in a randomised phase III study: 5-year analysis of the EORTC-NCIC trial. The lancet oncology. 2009 May;10(5):459–66.

[41] Ujifuku K, Mitsutake N, Takakura S, Matsuse M, Saenko V, Suzuki K, et al. miR-195, miR-455-3p and miR-10a(*) are implicated in acquired temozolomide resistance in glioblastomamultiforme cells. Cancer letters. 2010 Oct 28;296(2):241–8.

[42] Slaby O, Lakomy R, Fadrus P, Hrstka R, Kren L, Lzicarova E, et al. MicroRNA-181 family predicts response to concomitant chemoradiotherapy with temozolomide in glioblastoma patients. Neoplasma. 2010 Jan;57(3):264–9.

[43] Li Y, Li W, Yang Y, Lu Y, He C, Hu G, et al. MicroRNA-21 targets LRRFIP1 and contributes to VM-26 resistance in glioblastomamultiforme. Brain research. 2009 Aug 25;1286:13–8.

[44] Ren Y, Zhou X, Mei M, Yuan X-B, Han L, Wang G-X, et al. MicroRNA-21 inhibitor sensitizes human glioblastoma cells U251 (PTEN-mutant) and LN229 (PTEN-wild type) to taxol. BMC cancer. 2010 Jan;10:27.

[45] McElhinney RS, McMurry TBH, Margison GP. O6-alkylguanine-DNA alkyltransferase inactivation in cancer chemotherapy. Mini reviews in medicinal chemistry. 2003 Aug;3(5):471–85.

[46] Sullivan JM. Estrogen replacement therapy. The American Journal of Medicine. 1996 Oct;101(4):56S–60S.

[47] Ferrara N, Hillan KJ, Novotny W. Bevacizumab (Avastin), a humanized anti-VEGF monoclonal antibody for cancer therapy. Biochemical and biophysical research communications. 2005 Jul 29;333(2):328–35.

[48] Costanzo R, Piccirillo MC, Sandomenico C, Carillio G, Montanino A, Daniele G, et al. Gefitinib in non small cell lung cancer. Journal of biomedicine & biotechnology. 2011 Jan;2011:815269.

[49] Capdeville R, Buchdunger E, Zimmermann J, Matter A. Glivec (STI571, imatinib), a rationally developed, targeted anticancer drug. Nature reviews. Drug discovery. 2002 Jul;1(7):493–502.

[50] Rao SAM, Santosh V, Somasundaram K. Genome-wide expression profiling identifies deregulated miRNAs in malignant astrocytoma. Modern pathology: an official journal of the United States and Canadian Academy of Pathology, Inc. 2010 Oct; 23(10):1404–17.

[51] Parsons DW, Jones S, Zhang X, Lin JC-H, Leary RJ, Angenendt P, et al. An integrated genomic analysis of human glioblastomamultiforme. Science (New York, N.Y.). 2008 Sep 26;321(5897):1807–12.

[52] Elmén J, Thonberg H, Ljungberg K, Frieden M, Westergaard M, Xu Y, et al. Locked nucleic acid (LNA) mediated improvements in siRNA stability and functionality. Nucleic acids research. 2005 Jan;33(1):439–47.

[53] Soutschek J, Akinc A, Bramlage B, Charisse K, Constien R, Donoghue M, et al. Therapeutic silencing of an endogenous gene by systemic administration of modified siRNAs. Nature. 2004 Nov 11;432(7014):173–8.

[54] Corey DR. Chemical modification: the key to clinical application of RNA interference? The Journal of clinical investigation. 2007 Dec;117(12):3615–22.

[55] Whitehead K a, Langer R, Anderson DG. Knocking down barriers: advances in siR-NA delivery. Nature reviews. Drug discovery. 2009 Feb;8(2):129–38.

[56] Lee JB, Hong J, Bonner DK, Poon Z, Hammond PT. Self-assembled RNA interference microsponges for efficient siRNA delivery. Nature materials. 2012 Apr;11(4):316–22.

[57] Tao Y, Ruan J, Yeh S-H, Lu X, Wang Y, Zhai W, et al. Rapid growth of a hepatocellu-lar carcinoma and the driving mutations revealed by cell-population genetic analysis of whole-genome data. Proceedings of the National Academy of Sciences of the Unit-ed States of America. 2011 Jul 19;108(29):12042–7.

[58] Puente XS, Pinyol M, Quesada V, Conde L, Ordóñez GR, Villamor N, et al. Whole-genome sequencing identifies recurrent mutations in chronic lymphocytic leukaemia. Nature. 2011 Jul 7;475(7354):101–5.

[59] Stephens PJ, Tarpey PS, Davies H, Van Loo P, Greenman C, Wedge DC, et al. The landscape of cancer genes and mutational processes in breast cancer. Nature. 2012 Jun 21;486(7403):400–4.

Pediatric Brain Tumors

Chapter 5

New Molecular Targets and Treatments for Pediatric Brain Tumors

Claudia C. Faria, Christian A. Smith and
James T. Rutka

Additional information is available at the end of the chapter

1. Introduction

The outstanding progress in advanced molecular technologies has provided a tremendous amount of data that has altered the way in which we classify and categorize pediatric brain tumors. From the initial identification of chromosomal aberrations by karyotyping and comparative genomic hybridization, we have rapidly moved to expression array studies and to integrative genomic approaches which allowed the stratification of several pediatric brain tumors into molecular subgroups. These data have not only increased our understanding of the molecular pathogenesis of pediatric brain tumors, but have also identified prognostic markers and opened new avenues for targeted therapies.

One of the most important discoveries in pediatric astrocytomas was the duplication and the mutation of the v-raf murine sarcoma viral oncogene homolog B1 *(BRAF)* gene, found in pilocytic astrocytomas and malignant astrocytomas, respectively. Clinical trials using BRAF signaling pathway inhibitors are currently ongoing.

Until recently, the biology of diffuse intrinsic pontine glioma (DIPG) was poorly understood. Overexpression of epidermal growth factor receptor *(EGFR)* and platelet-derived growth factor receptor alpha *(PDGFRα)* amplification have now been reported in multiple studies in DIPG and clinical trials with the respective inhibitors (nimotuzumab for *EGFR* and dasatinib for PDGFRα), alone or in combination with other drugs, are in progress.

Integrated genomics has shown that medulloblastoma, the most common malignant pediatric brain tumor, comprises four distinct molecular and clinical variants. The stratification of patients into the Wnt subgroup, the sonic hedgehog (SHH) subgroup, Group 3 and Group 4 may lead to the identification of those patients that will most likely benefit from targeted therapies, like SMO inhibitors. Moreover, this molecular classification may help identify patients predicted to have a poor prognosis, who may benefit from intensified therapies, and patients with a favorable prognosis that potentially benefit from reduced radiation and chemotherapy regimens. It is already known from four independent studies that the Wnt subgroup patients have a very good prognosis while patients in Group 3 have a high incidence of metastasis and a dismal prognosis.

The transcriptional profiling of two large independent cohorts of posterior fossa ependymomas also identified two groups with distinct molecular and clinical features. Group A ependymomas have a balanced genome, occur in younger patients and tumors are located laterally. These patients have a worse clinical outcome and higher incidence of metastasis and recurrence. In contrast, Group B ependymomas occur in the midline and have a better prognosis. Since ependymomas are usually refractory to current chemotherapeutic agents, these discoveries may shed some light into the pathways involved in tumor initiation and progression and also identify new targets for therapy.

We are now facing the next-generation (Next-Gen) sequencing era which will provide further insights into the dysregulated signaling pathways in each tumor type. The identification of driver mutations will allow a better understanding of tumorigenesis and lead to the development of more accurate preclinical models. Moreover, the profiling of transcriptomes, genetic and epigenetic events of large cohorts of tumors will eventually shed some light into the cells of origin of specific subgroups and also the important driver events for tumor initiation, maintenance and progression. On the clinical side, this knowledge will allow the stratification of patients into appropriate risk groups and the tailoring of treatments according to each tumor's genomic landscape. In this chapter we describe the latest advances in molecular genomics of the most common pediatric brain tumors as well as its prognostic significance and relevance to the clinic. We also highlight the most recent clinical trials using molecular targeted therapies and discuss further possible avenues in the treatment of pediatric brain cancer.

2. Astrocytomas

Astrocytomas are a common brain tumor in children. According to the 2007 classification of the World Health Organization (WHO) they can be classified into four grades (WHO grade I-IV), which reflect their biological and clinical behavior. Pilocytic astrocytomas (WHO grade I) represent the most frequent brain tumor in the pediatric population and have excellent survival rates over 95% [1]. On the other hand, glioblastomas (WHO grade IV) are aggressive tumors, often non-responsive to treatments and with survival rates ranging from 10% to 30% [1]. We will focus on the molecular biology of these two types of pediatric astrocytomas.

2.1. Pilocytic astrocytoma

The first-line treatment for pilocytic astrocytoma (PA) is surgical resection. Although most children with these tumors survive for a long time, some will experience tumor recurrence, especially if the tumor resection is incomplete. Recurrent and progressive tumors are treated with radiation and/or chemotherapy but, until recently, the mechanisms of recurrence and malignant transformation were poorly understood.

Early studies on chromosomal aberrations in PAs showed normal karyotypes in most cases. Trisomy of chromosomes 5 and 7 and 7q gains were some of the few cytogenetic abnormalities found [2]. Using an array-based comparative genomic hybridization (array-CGH), Pfister *et al.* studied a large series of pediatric low-grade astrocytomas and uncovered mechanisms of mitogen-activated protein kinase (MAPK) activation in these tumors. The authors identified a tandem duplication of the *BRAF* gene locus (7q34) in more than 50% of the PAs and, in a smaller percentage (~6%) of tumors, a *BRAF* activating mutation V600E (a valine to glutamate change at hotspot codon 600) [3]. Later, it was demonstrated that the constitutive activation of BRAF was due to a fusion between a novel gene *(KIAA1549)* and the *BRAF* oncogene and also that this fusion was related to a better clinical outcome in incompletely resected low-grade astrocytomas [4]. Other, less frequent, reported gene fusions in PAs include the fusion of *BRAF* with the *FAM131B* gene and the fusion between a Raf kinase family member *(RAF1)* and SLIT-ROBO Rho GTPase-activating protein 3 *(SRGAP3)* gene [5]. The combined analysis of *BRAF* and isocitrate dehydrogenase 1 *(IDH1)* was shown to be both sensitive and specific to separate PAs from diffuse astrocytomas (WHO grade II). PAs contained the *KIAA1549:BRAF* fusion in 70% of cases but no *IDH2* or *IDH2* mutations while diffuse astrocytomas exhibited 76% of cases with *IDH1* mutations but no *BRAF* fusion [6]. There is also an interesting correlation between tumor location and the type of MAPK alteration. Posterior fossa tumors usually have increased incidence of *KIAA1549:BRAF* fusion while supratentorial tumors have high frequency of *BRAF*^{V600E} mutation. Approximately 80-90% of PA cases reported in the literature have at least one alteration in the MAPK pathway. Interestingly, all the alterations described in the MAPK pathway seem to be mutually exclusive suggesting that a single hit may be sufficient to induce transformation [5].

With the discovery of constitutive activation of MAPK pathway and BRAF alterations in most PAs, there has been an increasing interest in using these targets for novel therapeutic approaches. A number of phase I and phase II clinical trials are ongoing to test small molecule inhibitors of MAPK and related pathways (Table 1).

Drug		Clinical Trial	Reference (http://clinicaltrials.gov)
Group	Name		
MEK inhibitor	AZD6244	Phase I	NCT01386450, NCT01089101
RAF inhibitor (multikinase inhibitor)	Sorafenib	Phase II	NCT01338857 (suspended)
mTOR inhibitor	Everolimus	Phase II	NCT01158651, NCT00782626

Table 1. Pediatric clinical trials for pilocytic astrocytomas using targeted therapies

2.2. Glioblastoma multiforme

Glioblastoma multiforme (GBM) is the most common brain tumor in adults and is less fre-quent in the pediatric population. Despite improvements in neurosurgery and neuro-oncol-ogy, children diagnosed with GBM still have a dismal outcome with low survival rates even with aggressive therapeutic regimens. Although the histology of pediatric and adult GBMs appears identical, the molecular biology of these tumors is different. Therefore, the develop-ment of effective therapies for GBM in children should probably not rely on advances made in adult tumors.

Mutations in phosphatase and tensin homolog (*PTEN*) and amplifications of *EGFR* are com-mon in adult malignant gliomas but less frequent in the pediatric setting. However, when compared to pediatric low-grade gliomas, pediatric GBMs have a significant higher expres-sion of *EGFR*, although with no reported mutations and few deletions (~17%) in *EGFRvIII* [7]. While in adult GBMs the activation of the AKT pathway is a result of *PTEN* mutations, in pediatric tumors these are infrequent, although overexpression of AKT and its association with poor survival has been reported [8,9]. In a study with a large cohort of pediatric high-grade gliomas (HGGs) (37 GBMs out of 63 tumor samples), Bax *et al.* identified *PDGFRα* amplification and cyclin-dependent kinase inhibitor 2A/B (*CDKN2A/B*) deletion as the most frequent focal events. Interestingly, the patients with high-grade tumors and a stable ge-nomic profile had a better survival, independent of the histological grade or type [10]. Sever-al studies showed that *IDH1* mutations, common in adult secondary GBM (98%), are rare in pediatric GBM [7]. *TP53* (tumor protein 53) mutations were reported in pediatric high-grade tumors with an increased frequency in older children (40%) when compared to those less than 3 years (12%) [11]. Overexpression of p53, but not *TP53* mutations, was also associated with a significant reduction in the 5 year progression-free survival [12]. A recent study used high resolution single nucleotide polymorphism (SNP) arrays to identify novel chromoso-mal alterations in pediatric GBM, including amplifications of 7q21-22 and 1q43-44 and loss of heterozygosity (LOH) in15q15.1-15q23 and 17p13-17p11.2. Genes involved in cell-cycle regulation and cell death pathways were the predominant targets of LOHs [13].

It has been shown that overexpression of O^6-methylguanine-DNA methyltransferase (MGMT) is rare in HGGs but it has also been reported that it is associated with a poor over-all survival in children. The *MGMT* gene encodes a DNA-repair enzyme that can reduce the efficacy of alkylating agents. When the *MGMT* gene is silenced by promoter methylation, DNA repair in tumor tissue is compromised and patients have a better survival [7].

Finaly, a very recent study uncovered an interesting interplay between genetic and epige-netic events in pediatric GBM. The authors performed whole-exome sequencing in 48 pedia-tric GBMs and identified 44% of tumors harbouring somatic mutations in genes involved in the chromatin remodeling pathway, including the histone H3 gene (*H3F3A*), the α-thalassae-mia/mental retardation syndrome X-linked (*ATRX*) gene and the death-domain associated protein (*DAXX*) gene [14]. Interestingly, the *H3F3A* mutations were found to be specific of GBMs and more prevalent in the pediatric population. Moreover, 54% of all cases and 86% of patients with *H3F3A* and/or *ATRX* mutations, also showed *TP53* somatic mutations [14].

The novel targeted therapies that are currently under clinical investigation for high-grade gliomas, including GBM, are reviewed in reference [15].

3. Diffuse intrinsic pontine glioma

Despite decades of clinical research, the prognosis of diffuse intrinsic pontine glioma (DIPG) remains dismal with more than 90% of affected children dying within two years of diagnosis [16]. The only known effective treatment is radiation therapy although in most patients it has a transient effect. Different combinations of chemotherapy, radiation and radiosensitizers were attempted but failed to improve long-term survival [17]. The indication for biopsy in DIPG has been reserved for atypical tumors (prominent enhancement in magnetic ressonance imaging (MRI), low T2/FLAIR signal and/or high signal on diffuse imaging). However, the recognition that it is crucial to understand the biology of DIPG in order to design more rational drug treatments, led to a plea for routine biopsies in these patients. Some groups are already performing regular image-guided stereotactic biopsies in patients with DIPGs [18,19] and, furthermore, biopsies have been included in a clinical trial to decide which patients with DIPG would benefit from targeted therapy with erlotinib, an *EGFR* inhibitor [20]. Autopsies became another important source of DIPG tissue collection. Recent studies showed that up to 50% of parents agree with the autopsy and, if done within a short period of time after death, it is possible to obtain good quality DNA and RNA and even culture primary DIPG cell lines [21-23].

The paradigm shift to obtain tissue from patients with DIPG not only increased our knowledge in the molecular biology of the disease but also raised important clinical considerations. Paugh *et al.* described differences at the copy number and expression level in both adult and pediatric HGGs, including DIPGs. They showed that gain of chromosome 1q and *PDGFRα* amplification were frequent in children while chromosome 7 gain, 10q loss and *EGFR* amplification were characteristic of adult HGGs [24]. The identification of these two distinct biological entities has important clinical implications since pediatric clinical trials over the past decades have been designed with drugs known to have some activity in adult HGGs. It is now clear that DIPG has to be considered and treated as a separate disease. The same group compared the copy number alterations (CNAs) in DIPGs and nonbrainstem pediatric glioblastomas concluding that they are also genomically distinct. They identified receptor tyrosine kinase and retinoblastoma protein (*RB*) amplifications in 47% and 30% of DIPG cases, respectively, and found high frequency of focal amplifications of *PDGFRα, MET* and insuline-like growth factor receptor 1 *(IGF1R)* [25]. Furthermore, Zarghooni *et al.,* using SNP arrays, showed that DIPGs have distinct CNAs from pediatric supratentorial high-grade astrocytomas, with gains in *PDGFRα* and poly (ADP-ribose) polymerase-1 *(PARP-1)* amongst the most frequent [26]. Another group showed other differences between these tumors including frequent losses of 17p and 14q in DIPGs [27]. A very recent study used DNA from tumor tissue obtained at diagnosis by steriotactic biopsies and identified oncogenic mutations in *TP53* (40%), *PI3KCA* (15%) and *ATM/MPL* (5%). In fact, *PI3KCA* represents the first mutated oncogene described in DIPG [28].

Another level of gene expression regulation in DIPG occurs through epigenetic mechanisms, including histone modifications. Very recent sudies used whole-genome sequencing in large cohorts of DIPGs to identify somatic mutations in the *H3F3A* gene. Khuong-Quang *et al.* reported mutations in H3.3 that resulted in the substitution of lysine by methionine at amino acid 27 (K27M-H3.3) in 71% of cases and the presence of these mutations were associated with a worse survival independent of patient age and histological grade [29]. Furthermore, gains or amplifications in *PDGFRα* and *MYC/PVT1* were exclusively seen in K27M-H3.3 mutants. The authors also described *TP53* mutations in 77% and *ATRX* mutations in 9% of DIPGs [29]. Interestingly, both the mutated and wild-type H3.3 subgroups showed high frequency of *TP53* mutation. In another study, Wu *et al.* identified mutations in *H3F3A* (encodes histone H3.3) and *HIST1H3B* (encodes histone H3.1) in 78% of DIPGs and 22% of nonbrainstem pediatric glioblastomas [30]. The different H3 mutations were mutually exclusive and seemed to be a feature of pediatric HGGs.

The discoveries from the molecular biology of DIPGs identified several drugable targets allowing the development of molecular target-based trials that are summarized in Table 2. Some of these trials have shown a subset of patients with survival longer than expected and, therefore, several other trials are ongoing, some of them including combined therapies [17,31].

Finally, DIPG treatment involves another challenge which is drug distribution. Probably due to an intact blood-brain barrier, penetration of drugs in the pons seems to be poor, a fact demonstrated by the lack of gadolinium enhancement in the MRI in most DIPGs. Therefore, it is crucial to improve drug delivery either by disrupting the blood-brain barrier (e.g. focused ultrasound or drugs that increase permeability such as manitol), by local delivery (tumor injection or convection enhanced delivery) or even nanoparticles [17]. These techniques may promote high drug concentrations in the pons, including agents that normally don't cross the blood-brain barrier.

Drug	Clinical Trial	1 year Overall Survival (OS)	Reference
Imatinib	Phase I	45.5%	2007 [32]
Tipifarnib	Phase I	36.4%	2008 [33]
Gefitinib	Phase I	48%	2010 [34]
Vandetanib	Phase I	37%	2010 [35]
Erlotinib	Phase I	50%	2011 [20]
Gefitinib	Phase II	56%	2011 [36]
Nimotuzumab	Phase II	Median OS 9.6 months	2011 [37]

Table 2. Clinical trials for diffuse intrinsic pontine glioma (DIPG) using targeted therapies

4. Medulloblastoma

Medulloblastoma, the commonest malignant brain tumor in the pediatric population, is no longer considered a single disease. Recent efforts of multiple independent groups have reached to a consensus that medulloblastoma comprises four distinct molecular variants named WNT, SHH, Group 3 and Group 4 [38]. The subgroups have different demographics, genetic profiles and prognosis [39]. This may explain why patients with the same histological disease have different clinical outcomes and a variable response to current treatments including surgery, whole-brain radiation and intensive chemotherapy. Figure 1 summarizes the main features of the four medulloblastoma subgroups.

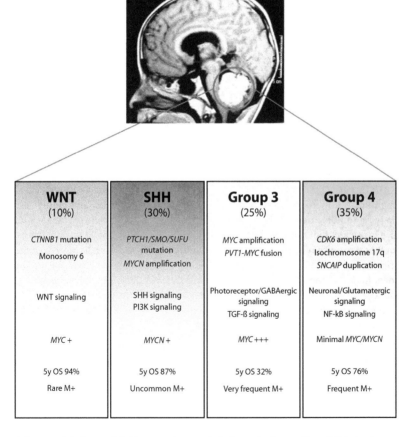

WNT (10%)	SHH (30%)	Group 3 (25%)	Group 4 (35%)
CTNNB1 mutation Monosomy 6	PTCH1/SMO/SUFU mutation MYCN amplification	MYC amplification PVT1-MYC fusion	CDK6 amplification Isochromosome 17q SNCAIP duplication
WNT signaling	SHH signaling PI3K signaling	Photoreceptor/GABAergic signaling TGF-ß signaling	Neuronal/Glutamatergic signaling NF-kB signaling
MYC +	MYCN +	MYC +++	Minimal MYC/MYCN
5y OS 94%	5y OS 87%	5y OS 32%	5y OS 76%
Rare M+	Uncommon M+	Very frequent M+	Frequent M+

Figure 1. Features of the four medulloblastoma subgroups, including molecular genetics and clinical outcome

4.1. WNT medulloblastomas

WNT medulloblastomas are frequent in older children and teenagers and are rarely seen in infants. Patients within this subgroup have usually an excellent outcome with survival rates over 90%. However, Remke *et al.* showed that this is only true for pediatric cases as adult WNT patients exhibit survival rates of approximately 80% [40]. Histologically, WNT tumors are almost always of the classic variant and they rarely disseminate.

This subgroup is enriched in genes of the WNT pathway. Although few gains and losses were reported in the WNT genome, mutations in *CTNNB1* are frequent and usually occur with deletion of one copy of chromosome 6 (monosomy 6). Patients with *CTNNB1* mutation have accumulation of β-catenin in the nucleus and better survival rates. Positive nuclear immunostaining for β-catenin is now currently accepted as a marker of WNT medulloblastomas [41,42], although DKK1 and DKK2 were also proposed as markers for this subgroup [42,43]. The overall good outcome of WNT tumors suggests that this subgroup may be a good candidate for de-escalation therapy in future clinical trials.

4.2. SHH medulloblastomas

SHH medulloblastomas are frequently found in infants and adults (approximately 60% of cases in each age group) but are rare in childhood. In the SHH subgroup, prognostic factors such as M-stage and desmoplasia are age-dependent. Metastasis at presentation represents a negative prognostic factor only in adults while desmoplasia is associated with worse outcome only in pediatric cases [44]. From a histological point of view this subgroup is unique since it includes tumors of the four main variants (classic, nodular desmoplastic, large-cell anaplastic and medulloblastoma with extensive nodularity).

SHH medulloblastomas are characterized by aberrant expression of SHH pathway genes including *SMO, PTCH1, SUFU* and *GLI2*. Amplifications of *MYCN* and *YAP1* are also seen in this subgroup. Additionally, deletion of chromosome 9q is a common and highly restricted event in SHH tumors, most likely secondary to *PTCH1* mutation on chromosome 9q22 [45]. Of notice is the fact that the transcriptomes of pediatric and adult SHH tumors have different expression profiles with increased levels of genes related to extracellular matrix function in the first group and elevated levels of *HOX* family genes and genes involved in tissue development in the second group [44,46]. In an attempt to simplify the molecular subgrouping of medulloblastomas, different laboratories used formalin-fixed paraffin-embedded tissues (FFPE) to test a variety of markers for SHH medulloblastomas including SFRP1, GLI1 and GAB1 [42,43,47].

The clinical and molecular distinction of infant and adult SHH medulloblastomas suggests a disparate underlying biology and raises the question of possible different responses to current targeted therapies.

4.3. Group 3 medulloblastomas

Group 3 medulloblastomas are restricted to pediatric patients. Indeed, two recent studies concluded that Group 3 tumors are extremely rare in adults [40,48]. Another feature of this subgroup is its aggressive behavior with high incidence of metastasis, frequent large-cell anaplastic histology and an invariable dismal prognosis (approximately 20 to 30% overall survival). It has been shown that Group 3 medulloblastomas consist of two distinct subtypes one of which harbors frequent amplifications of the *MYC* gene and has the worse outcome [49]. Although Group 3 and 4 have some common genetic features, including gain of chromosome 7, losses of chromosomes 5q and 10q and gain of chromosome 1q are more frequent in Group 3 tumors. NPR3 and KCNA1 were proposed as biomarkers for Group 3 and Group 4, respectively [42].

Until recently, there were no known targetable pathways in Group 3 medulloblastomas and the suggested intensification of treatment for these patients would necessarily result in increased toxicity and morbidity (see below).

4.4. Group 4 medulloblastomas

Group 4 tumors represent simultaneously the most common and the less well-understood subgroup of medulloblastomas. They are found across all age groups and have an intermediate prognosis although the adult patients show a reduced survival when compared to their pediatric counterparts. Group 4 medulloblastomas are usually of the classic variant and they rarely present with metastasis. The most frequent genetic aberration in Group 4 tumors, present in up to 80% of cases, is isochromosome 17q (i17q) although *MYCN* amplifications were also reported. The expression of follistatin-related protein 5 (*FSTL5*) was identified as a marker of high-risk Group 4 patients [50].

4.5. From genomic revolution to clinical trials in medulloblastoma

Despite important advances in medulloblastoma treatment, approximately 40% of children will have recurrence and 30% will die from the disease. Moreover, the survivors are often left with significant disabilities due to cytotoxic side effects of chemotherapy and radiation to the developing central nervous system (CNS). Identifying the genetic events that drive medulloblastoma is, therefore, critical to develop more effective and less toxic therapies.

Except for SHH inhibitors that have shown some promise in SHH patients [51], there were no other targetable genes or pathways for WNT, Group 3 and Group 4 medulloblastomas. However, very recently published studies from four independent groups dissected the genomic landscape of medulloblastoma using large cohorts of patients and the latest high-throughput technology.

Using SNP arrays in a large cohort of over 1,000 medulloblastoma samples, Northcott *et al.* reported that somatic CNAs are a common event in medulloblastoma and are subgroup-specific [52]. In Group 3 tumors the authors identified recurrent *PVT1* gene fusions with *MYC* and *NDRG1* through chromothripsis, a process of erroneous DNA repair after chromosome shattering. This process of catastrophic DNA rearrangement has been previously shown in SHH medulloblastomas with *TP53* mutations [53]. The most frequent somatic CNA was a duplication of *SNCAIP*, a gene on chromosome 5q23.2 involved in Parkinson's disease. Interestingly, *SNCAIP* duplication is restricted to Group 4α, a subtype of Group 4 with a relatively balanced genome when compared to Group 4β [52]. The authors also reported novel targetable pathways that could be the basis for future clinical trials, including PI3K pathway in SHH, TGF-β pathway in Group 3 and NF-κB pathway in Group 4 [52].

Another interesting observation, consistent with the first published study using genome sequencing in medulloblastoma [54], is the low number of somatic mutations found in these tumors when compared to adult solid tumors and the increased mutation frequency with age [52,55-57]. Jones *et al.* also identified tetraploidy as an early event in Group 3 and Group 4 medulloblastomas, concomitant with *TP53* mutations in some tumors [55].

The genome sequencing of independent cohorts of medulloblastoma samples and matched blood, identified previously known mutated genes (*CTNNB1, PTCH1, MLL2, SMARCA4, TP53*) but also allowed the discovery of new recurrent somatic mutations (*DDX3X, CTDNEP1, KDM6A, TBR1, GPS2, BCOR, LDB1, EZH2, CHD7, ZMYM3*), often subgroup-specific [52,55-57]. Notably, these studies identified genes involved in histone modification and chromatin remodeling complexes across all subgroups, which may explain the complexity and heterogeneity seen in medulloblastoma.

The ongoing genomic revolution in medulloblastoma is moving the next generation of clinical trials towards targeted treatments according to the molecular subgroup. SHH inhibitors, including GDC-0449 and NVP-LDE225, already proved its efficacy in tumor growth reduction but the reported acquired resistance suggests that a combination of targeted therapies may be a key approach to improve response [58]. Phase II clinical trials using GDC-0449 are now recruiting pediatric and adult patients with recurrent or refractory medulloblastoma and phase I trials with NVP-LDE225 are recruiting patients with advanced solid tumors including medulloblastoma. Under debate is the de-escalation of therapy in WNT patients and the intensification of treatment and/or targeted therapy for Group 3 patients [59,60]. Finaly, the discovery of a significant number of chromatin modifier genes across medulloblastoma subgroups suggests that histone deacetylase inhibitors may constitute a good therapeutic option in the future.

5. Ependymoma

Ependymoma, the third most common brain tumor in childhood, is still incurable in up to 45% of patients [61]. The gold standard of treatment is maximal safe surgical resection followed by radiation since chemotherapy is usually ineffective. Ependymomas can arise in different regions of the CNS including the cerebral hemispheres, the posterior fossa and the spinal cord. This diversity is extended to its demographic, genetic, clinical and prognostic characteristics. Both children and adults can be affected although posterior fossa tumors are more common in children and supratentorial and spinal tumors occur more frequently in adults. The clinical behavior of ependymoma is variable with some patients experiencing a fatal clinical course while others have a long recurrence-free survival. The lack of novel targeted treatments for ependymoma can be explained by the paucity of cell lines and animal models of the disease.

The genetic heterogeneity of ependymoma has been highlighted by different studies with some cohorts of tumors showing frequent chromosomal alterations and others displaying a balanced genome. Korshunov *et al.* identified gain of chromosome 1q, *CDKN2A* homozygous deletion and age at diagnosis as independent factors of worse prognosis in ependymoma [62]. Johnson *et al.* described subgroups of ependymoma clustered by their CNAs, messenger RNA (mRNA) and microRNA (miRNA) profiles and, interestingly, tumors were segregated by their CNS location [63]. Furthermore, the authors were able to generate a mouse model of supratentorial ependymoma presenting strong evidence that the radial glial cells are likely the cells of origin of this tumor [63]. More recently, Witt *et al.* transcriptionaly profiled two large independent cohorts of posterior fossa tumors identifying two distinct subgroups, Group A and Group B ependymomas [64]. Group A tumors comprise only posterior fossa ependymomas while Group B tumors include posterior fossa tumors that clustered with spinal ependymomas. Patients with Group A ependymomas are younger (median age 2.5 years), with the majority of tumors located laterally and with a balanced genome. These patients have higher incidence of recurrence and metastasis and a worse prognosis (5 year overall survival of 69%). Patients with Group B ependymomas are older (median age 20 years), with tumors in the midline (95%) and a high degree of genomic instability (Figure 2). Although several cytogenetic abnormalities were found in this group, including loss of chromosomes 1, 2, 3, 6, 8, 10, 14q, 17q, 22q, and gain of chromosomes 4, 5q, 7, 9, 11, 12, 15q, 18, 20, and 21q, patients have a good prognosis (5 year overall survival of 95%). The genes that characterize Group B ependymomas are involved in microtubule assembly and oxidative metabolism while Group A tumors include several pathways associated with cancer. The authors identified *LAMA2* and *NELL2* as markers of Group A and Group B ependymomas, respectively [64]. Using unsupervised cluster analysis of gene expression signatures, others also described two groups of infratentorial ependymomas (Group 1 and Group 2) that overlap with Group A and Group B of Witt *et al.*, respectively [65]. The distinct genetic profiles of posterior fossa ependymomas suggest that novel targeted therapies against subgroup-specific pathways maybe the key strategy to improve survival, particularly in Group A patients.

The interesting observation that up to 50% of pediatric ependymomas have a balanced genome [62] raises the possibility that epigenetic mechanisms may play a role in ependymoma pathogenesis. Most studies have focused on promoter hypermethylation of candidate genes known to be tumor suppressor genes in ependymoma or frequently methylated in other cancers. *HIC-1* and *RASSF1A* promoter hypermethylation were described in 83% and 86% of ependymomas, respectively. They are known to be tumor suppressor genes, silenced by hypermethylation in many human cancers [66]. Promoter hypermethylation of other genes, including *CDKN2A* (21%), *CDKN2B* (32%), *p14ARF* (21%), and *MGMT* (27%) were also reported in studies with large cohorts of tumor samples [66]. More recently, Rogers *et al.* used an array-based analysis to determine the methylation profile of 98 ependymomas [67]. The authors found that supratentorial and spinal ependymomas have a hypermethylated phenotype and that the genes identified are involved in cell growth and apoptosis. The increase in promoter methylation of CpG islands across a large number of genes has been described in other cancers as CpG island methylator phenotype (CIMP). Although it has been correlated to a worse outcome in other cancers, the authors could not find an association between methylation and prognosis in ependymomas [67].

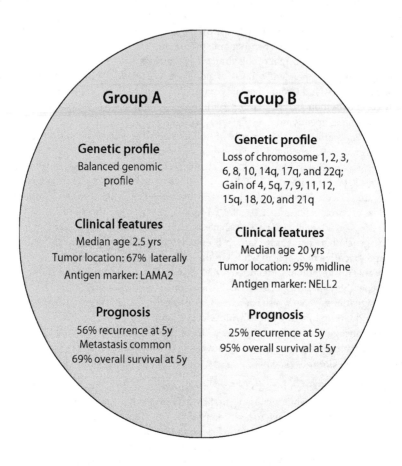

Figure 2. Features of the posterior fossa ependymoma subgroups, including genetic profile, clinical features and prognosis.

Another less frequent epigenetic event in cancer genomes is hypomethylation. This loss of DNA methylation occurs mainly in repetitive elements (Alu repeats). In a recent study, Xie *et al.* used a genome-wide approach to study the methylation profiles of Alu repeat sequences in pediatric intracranial ependymomas [68]. Notably, they identified a global loss of methylation in the regions flanking, rather than within, Alu sequences, and this was correlated with a more agressive tumor phenotype. The biological significance of this finding is yet to be unraveled.

The increased knowledge of the genetic and epigenetic events that drive ependymoma may lead to more effective targeted therapies aimed to repair molecular functions and dysregulated pathways. However, there are currently no clinical trials evaluating specific molecular therapies in ependymoma. Despite the recent achievements in ependymoma research, greater progress is needed to decifer the molecular and biological mechanisms of this disease and, ultimately, to improve patient's clinical outcome.

6. Conclusion

Major steps have been made to a better understanding of the molecular genetics underlying the most common pediatric brain tumors. An important advance was to recognize that adult and pediatric brain tumors are distinct and, therefore, need different therapeutic approaches. This knowledge opened new avenues for targeted therapies and clinical trials based on tumor-specific molecular subgrouping are currently ongoing. When compared to standard chemotherapy and radiation, the use of biological agents has several advantages. They can target cancer cells and spare normal cells in the developing CNS of children and also be used to delay radiotherapy, which is responsible for long-term side effects of treatment. Many of the newer agents are small molecules, with low molecular weight, which facilitates blood-brain barrier penetration. However, despite the enthusiasm with the phase I and phase II clinical trials using biological agents as monotherapy, mainly for progressive and recurrent brain tumors, efficacy has not yet been proven. In the future, combination therapies will likely be needed to target multiple pathways involved in tumorigenesis and to overcome the cytostatic effect of several biological agents. As the amount of data generated by high-throughput studies increases the drugable targets for each pediatric brain tumor, the number of clinical trials will continue to expand aiming a better control of the disease with less morbidity and extended survival.

Acknowledgments

Claudia Faria was supported by a fellowship from The Hospital for Sick Children Research Training Centre and the Garron Family Cancer Centre. She is a PhD candidate from The Programme for Advanced Medical Education, supported by Fundação Gulbenkian, Fundação Champalimaud, Ministério da Saúde e Fundação para a Ciência e Tecnologia, Portugal. This work was also supported by grants from the Canadian Cancer Society Research Institute (grant no. 019073), the Wiley fund, the Laurie Berman Fund for Brain Tumour Research, Pediatric Brain Tumour Foundation of the United States, and B.r.a.i.n.child.

Author details

Claudia C. Faria[1], Christian A. Smith[2] and James T. Rutka[1]

1 Division of Neurosurgery and Labatt Brain Tumour Research Centre, The Hospital for Sick Children, University of Toronto, Canada

2 Labatt Brain Tumour Research Centre, The Hospital for Sick Children, University of Toronto, Canada

References

[1] Ohgaki H, Kleihues P. Population-based studies on incidence, survival rates, and genetic alterations in astrocytic and oligodendroglial gliomas. J Neuropathol Exp Neurol. 2005 Jun;64(6):479-89.

[2] Dubuc AM, Northcott PA, Mack S, Witt H, Pfister S, Taylor MD. The genetics of pediatric brain tumors. Curr Neurol Neurosci Rep. 2010 May;10(3):215-23.

[3] Pfister S, Janzarik WG, Remke M, Ernst A, Werft W, Becker N, et al. BRAF gene duplication constitutes a mechanism of MAPK pathway activation in low-grade astrocytomas. J Clin Invest. 2008 May;118(5):1739-49.

[4] Hawkins C, Walker E, Mohamed N, Zhang C, Jacob K, Shirinian M, et al. BRAF-KIAA1549 fusion predicts better clinical outcome in pediatric low-grade astrocytoma. Clin Cancer Res. 2011 Jul 15;17(14):4790-8.

[5] Jones DT, Gronych J, Lichter P, Witt O, Pfister SM. MAPK pathway activation in pilocytic astrocytoma. Cell Mol Life Sci. 2012 Jun;69(11):1799-811.

[6] Korshunov A, Meyer J, Capper D, Christians A, Remke M, Witt H, et al. Combined molecular analysis of BRAF and IDH1 distinguishes pilocytic astrocytoma from diffuse astrocytoma. Acta Neuropathol. 2009 Sep;118(3):401-5.

[7] MacDonald TJ, Aguilera D, Kramm CM. Treatment of high-grade glioma in children and adolescents. Neuro Oncol. 2011 Oct;13(10):1049-58.

[8] Faury D, Nantel A, Dunn SE, Guiot MC, Haque T, Hauser P, et al. Molecular profiling identifies prognostic subgroups of pediatric glioblastoma and shows increased YB-1 expression in tumors. J Clin Oncol. 2007 Apr 1;25(10):1196-208.

[9] Pollack IF, Hamilton RL, Burger PC, Brat DJ, Rosenblum MK, Murdoch GH, et al. Akt activation is a common event in pediatric malignant gliomas and a potential adverse prognostic marker: a report from the Children's Oncology Group. J Neurooncol. 2010 Sep;99(2):155-63.

[10] Bax DA, Mackay A, Little SE, Carvalho D, Viana-Pereira M, Tamber N, et al. A distinct spectrum of copy number aberrations in pediatric high-grade gliomas. Clin Cancer Res. 2010 Jul 1;16(13):3368-77.

[11] Pollack IF, Finkelstein SD, Burnham J, Holmes EJ, Hamilton RL, Yates AJ, et al. Age and TP53 mutation frequency in childhood malignant gliomas: results in a multi-institutional cohort. Cancer Res. 2001 Oct 15;61(20):7404-7.

[12] Pollack IF, Finkelstein SD, Woods J, Burnham J, Holmes EJ, Hamilton RL, et al. Expression of p53 and prognosis in children with malignant gliomas. N Engl J Med. 2002 Feb 7;346(6):420-7.

[13] Qu HQ, Jacob K, Fatet S, Ge B, Barnett D, Delattre O, et al. Genome-wide profiling using single-nucleotide polymorphism arrays identifies novel chromosomal imbalances in pediatric glioblastomas. Neuro Oncol. 2010 Feb;12(2):153-63.

[14] Schwartzentruber J, Korshunov A, Liu XY, Jones DT, Pfaff E, Jacob K, et al. Driver mutations in histone H3.3 and chromatin remodelling genes in paediatric glioblastoma. Nature. 2012 Feb 9;482(7384):226-31.

[15] Nageswara Rao AA, Scafidi J, Wells EM, Packer RJ. Biologically targeted therapeutics in pediatric brain tumors. Pediatr Neurol. 2012 Apr;46(4):203-11.

[16] Hargrave D, Bartels U, Bouffet E. Diffuse brainstem glioma in children: critical review of clinical trials. Lancet Oncol. 2006 Mar;7(3):241-8.

[17] Jansen MH, van Vuurden DG, Vandertop WP, Kaspers GJ. Diffuse intrinsic pontine gliomas: a systematic update on clinical trials and biology. Cancer Treat Rev. 2012 Feb;38(1):27-35.

[18] Roujeau T, Machado G, Garnett MR, Miquel C, Puget S, Geoerger B, et al. Stereotactic biopsy of diffuse pontine lesions in children. J Neurosurg. 2007 Jul;107(1 Suppl):1-4.

[19] Pirotte BJ, Lubansu A, Massager N, Wikler D, Goldman S, Levivier M. Results of positron emission tomography guidance and reassessment of the utility of and indications for stereotactic biopsy in children with infiltrative brainstem tumors. J Neurosurg. 2007 Nov;107(5 Suppl):392-9.

[20] Geoerger B, Hargrave D, Thomas F, Ndiaye A, Frappaz D, Andreiuolo F, et al. Innovative Therapies for Children with Cancer pediatric phase I study of erlotinib in brainstem glioma and relapsing/refractory brain tumors. Neuro Oncol. 2011 Jan; 13(1):109-18.

[21] Angelini P, Hawkins C, Laperriere N, Bouffet E, Bartels U. Post mortem examinations in diffuse intrinsic pontine glioma: challenges and chances. J Neurooncol. 2011 Jan;101(1):75-81.

[22] Broniscer A, Baker JN, Baker SJ, Chi SN, Geyer JR, Morris EB, et al. Prospective collection of tissue samples at autopsy in children with diffuse intrinsic pontine glioma. Cancer. 2010 Oct 1;116(19):4632-7.

[23] Caretti V, Jansen MH, van Vuurden DG, Lagerweij T, Bugiani M, Horsman I, et al. Implementation of a Multi-Institutional Diffuse Intrinsic Pontine Glioma Autopsy Protocol and Characterization of a Primary Cell Culture. Neuropathol Appl Neurobiol. 2012 Jul 27.

[24] Paugh BS, Qu C, Jones C, Liu Z, Adamowicz-Brice M, Zhang J, et al. Integrated molecular genetic profiling of pediatric high-grade gliomas reveals key differences with the adult disease. J Clin Oncol. 2010 Jun 20;28(18):3061-8.

[25] Paugh BS, Broniscer A, Qu C, Miller CP, Zhang J, Tatevossian RG, et al. Genome-wide analyses identify recurrent amplifications of receptor tyrosine kinases and cell-cycle regulatory genes in diffuse intrinsic pontine glioma. J Clin Oncol. 2011 Oct 20;29(30):3999-4006.

[26] Zarghooni M, Bartels U, Lee E, Buczkowicz P, Morrison A, Huang A, et al. Whole-genome profiling of pediatric diffuse intrinsic pontine gliomas highlights platelet-derived growth factor receptor alpha and poly (ADP-ribose) polymerase as potential therapeutic targets. J Clin Oncol. 2010 Mar 10;28(8):1337-44.

[27] Barrow J, Adamowicz-Brice M, Cartmill M, MacArthur D, Lowe J, Robson K, et al. Homozygous loss of ADAM3A revealed by genome-wide analysis of pediatric high-grade glioma and diffuse intrinsic pontine gliomas. Neuro Oncol. 2011 Feb;13(2): 212-22.

[28] Grill J, Puget S, Andreiuolo F, Philippe C, MacConaill L, Kieran MW. Critical oncogenic mutations in newly diagnosed pediatric diffuse intrinsic pontine glioma. Pediatr Blood Cancer. 2012 Apr;58(4):489-91.

[29] Khuong-Quang DA, Buczkowicz P, Rakopoulos P, Liu XY, Fontebasso AM, Bouffet E, et al. K27M mutation in histone H3.3 defines clinically and biologically distinct subgroups of pediatric diffuse intrinsic pontine gliomas. Acta Neuropathol. 2012 Sep; 124(3):439-47.

[30] Wu G, Broniscer A, McEachron TA, Lu C, Paugh BS, Becksfort J, et al. Somatic histone H3 alterations in pediatric diffuse intrinsic pontine gliomas and non-brainstem glioblastomas. Nat Genet. 2012 Mar;44(3):251-3.

[31] Bartels U, Hawkins C, Vezina G, Kun L, Souweidane M, Bouffet E. Proceedings of the diffuse intrinsic pontine glioma (DIPG) Toronto Think Tank: advancing basic and translational research and cooperation in DIPG. J Neurooncol. 2011 Oct;105(1):119-25.

[32] Pollack IF, Jakacki RI, Blaney SM, Hancock ML, Kieran MW, Phillips P, et al. Phase I trial of imatinib in children with newly diagnosed brainstem and recurrent malignant gliomas: a Pediatric Brain Tumor Consortium report. Neuro Oncol. 2007 Apr; 9(2):145-60.

[33] Haas-Kogan DA, Banerjee A, Kocak M, Prados MD, Geyer JR, Fouladi M, et al. Phase I trial of tipifarnib in children with newly diagnosed intrinsic diffuse brainstem glioma. Neuro Oncol. 2008 Jun;10(3):341-7.

[34] Geyer JR, Stewart CF, Kocak M, Broniscer A, Phillips P, Douglas JG, et al. A phase I and biology study of gefitinib and radiation in children with newly diagnosed brain stem gliomas or supratentorial malignant gliomas. Eur J Cancer. 2010 Dec;46(18): 3287-93.

[35] Broniscer A, Baker JN, Tagen M, Onar-Thomas A, Gilbertson RJ, Davidoff AM, et al. Phase I study of vandetanib during and after radiotherapy in children with diffuse intrinsic pontine glioma. J Clin Oncol. 2010 Nov 1;28(31):4762-8.

[36] Pollack IF, Stewart CF, Kocak M, Poussaint TY, Broniscer A, Banerjee A, et al. A phase II study of gefitinib and irradiation in children with newly diagnosed brain-stem gliomas: a report from the Pediatric Brain Tumor Consortium. Neuro Oncol. 2011 Mar;13(3):290-7.

[37] Massimino M, Bode U, Biassoni V, Fleischhack G. Nimotuzumab for pediatric diffuse intrinsic pontine gliomas. Expert Opin Biol Ther. 2011 Feb;11(2):247-56.

[38] Taylor MD, Northcott PA, Korshunov A, Remke M, Cho YJ, Clifford SC, et al. Molecular subgroups of medulloblastoma: the current consensus. Acta Neuropathol. 2012 Apr;123(4):465-72.

[39] Northcott PA, Korshunov A, Pfister SM, Taylor MD. The clinical implications of medulloblastoma subgroups. Nat Rev Neurol. 2012 Jun;8(6):340-51.

[40] Remke M, Hielscher T, Northcott PA, Witt H, Ryzhova M, Wittmann A, et al. Adult medulloblastoma comprises three major molecular variants. J Clin Oncol. 2011 Jul 1;29(19):2717-23.

[41] Fattet S, Haberler C, Legoix P, Varlet P, Lellouch-Tubiana A, Lair S, et al. Beta-catenin status in paediatric medulloblastomas: correlation of immunohistochemical expression with mutational status, genetic profiles, and clinical characteristics. J Pathol. 2009 May;218(1):86-94.

[42] Northcott PA, Korshunov A, Witt H, Hielscher T, Eberhart CG, Mack S, et al. Medulloblastoma comprises four distinct molecular variants. J Clin Oncol. 2011 Apr 10;29(11):1408-14.

[43] Thompson MC, Fuller C, Hogg TL, Dalton J, Finkelstein D, Lau CC, et al. Genomics identifies medulloblastoma subgroups that are enriched for specific genetic alterations. J Clin Oncol. 2006 Apr 20;24(12):1924-31.

[44] Northcott PA, Hielscher T, Dubuc A, Mack S, Shih D, Remke M, et al. Pediatric and adult sonic hedgehog medulloblastomas are clinically and molecularly distinct. Acta Neuropathol. 2011 Aug;122(2):231-40.

[45] Northcott PA, Dubuc AM, Pfister S, Taylor MD. Molecular subgroups of medulloblastoma. Expert Rev Neurother. 2012 Jul;12(7):871-84.

[46] Al-Halabi H, Nantel A, Klekner A, Guiot MC, Albrecht S, Hauser P, et al. Preponderance of sonic hedgehog pathway activation characterizes adult medulloblastoma. Acta Neuropathol. 2011 Feb;121(2):229-39.

[47] Ellison DW, Dalton J, Kocak M, Nicholson SL, Fraga C, Neale G, et al. Medulloblastoma: clinicopathological correlates of SHH, WNT, and non-SHH/WNT molecular subgroups. Acta Neuropathol. 2011 Mar;121(3):381-96.

[48] Kool M, Korshunov A, Remke M, Jones DT, Schlanstein M, Northcott PA, et al. Molecular subgroups of medulloblastoma: an international meta-analysis of transcriptome, genetic aberrations, and clinical data of WNT, SHH, Group 3, and Group 4 medulloblastomas. Acta Neuropathol. 2012 Apr;123(4):473-84.

[49] Cho YJ, Tsherniak A, Tamayo P, Santagata S, Ligon A, Greulich H, et al. Integrative genomic analysis of medulloblastoma identifies a molecular subgroup that drives poor clinical outcome. J Clin Oncol. 2011 Apr 10;29(11):1424-30.

[50] Remke M, Hielscher T, Korshunov A, Northcott PA, Bender S, Kool M, et al. FSTL5 is a marker of poor prognosis in non-WNT/non-SHH medulloblastoma. J Clin Oncol. 2011 Oct 10;29(29):3852-61.

[51] Rudin CM, Hann CL, Laterra J, Yauch RL, Callahan CA, Fu L, et al. Treatment of medulloblastoma with hedgehog pathway inhibitor GDC-0449. N Engl J Med. 2009 Sep 17;361(12):1173-8.

[52] Northcott PA, Shih DJ, Peacock J, Garzia L, Morrissy AS, Zichner T, et al. Subgroup-specific structural variation across 1,000 medulloblastoma genomes. Nature. 2012 Aug 2;488(7409):49-56.

[53] Rausch T, Jones DT, Zapatka M, Stutz AM, Zichner T, Weischenfeldt J, et al. Genome sequencing of pediatric medulloblastoma links catastrophic DNA rearrangements with TP53 mutations. Cell. 2012 Jan 20;148(1-2):59-71.

[54] Parsons DW, Li M, Zhang X, Jones S, Leary RJ, Lin JC, et al. The genetic landscape of the childhood cancer medulloblastoma. Science. 2011 Jan 28;331(6016):435-9.

[55] Jones DT, Jager N, Kool M, Zichner T, Hutter B, Sultan M, et al. Dissecting the genomic complexity underlying medulloblastoma. Nature. 2012 Aug 2;488(7409):100-5.

[56] Pugh TJ, Weeraratne SD, Archer TC, Pomeranz Krummel DA, Auclair D, Bochicchio J, et al. Medulloblastoma exome sequencing uncovers subtype-specific somatic mutations. Nature. 2012 Aug 2;488(7409):106-10.

[57] Robinson G, Parker M, Kranenburg TA, Lu C, Chen X, Ding L, et al. Novel mutations target distinct subgroups of medulloblastoma. Nature. 2012 Aug 2;488(7409):43-8.

[58] Metcalfe C, de Sauvage FJ. Hedgehog fights back: mechanisms of acquired resistance against Smoothened antagonists. Cancer Res. 2011 Aug 1;71(15):5057-61.

[59] Ramaswamy V, Northcott PA, Taylor MD. FISH and chips: the recipe for improved prognostication and outcomes for children with medulloblastoma. Cancer Genet. 2011 Nov;204(11):577-88.

[60] Leary SE, Olson JM. The molecular classification of medulloblastoma: driving the next generation clinical trials. Curr Opin Pediatr. 2012 Feb;24(1):33-9.

[61] Merchant TE, Li C, Xiong X, Kun LE, Boop FA, Sanford RA. Conformal radiotherapy after surgery for paediatric ependymoma: a prospective study. Lancet Oncol. 2009 Mar;10(3):258-66.

[62] Korshunov A, Witt H, Hielscher T, Benner A, Remke M, Ryzhova M, et al. Molecular staging of intracranial ependymoma in children and adults. J Clin Oncol. 2010 Jul 1;28(19):3182-90.

[63] Johnson RA, Wright KD, Poppleton H, Mohankumar KM, Finkelstein D, Pounds SB, et al. Cross-species genomics matches driver mutations and cell compartments to model ependymoma. Nature. 2010 Jul 29;466(7306):632-6.

[64] Witt H, Mack SC, Ryzhova M, Bender S, Sill M, Isserlin R, et al. Delineation of two clinically and molecularly distinct subgroups of posterior fossa ependymoma. Cancer Cell. 2011 Aug 16;20(2):143-57.

[65] Wani K, Armstrong TS, Vera-Bolanos E, Raghunathan A, Ellison D, Gilbertson R, et al. A prognostic gene expression signature in infratentorial ependymoma. Acta Neuropathol. 2012 May;123(5):727-38.

[66] Dubuc AM, Mack S, Unterberger A, Northcott PA, Taylor MD. The epigenetics of brain tumors. Methods Mol Biol. 2012;863:139-53.

[67] Rogers HA, Kilday JP, Mayne C, Ward J, Adamowicz-Brice M, Schwalbe EC, et al. Supratentorial and spinal pediatric ependymomas display a hypermethylated phenotype which includes the loss of tumor suppressor genes involved in the control of cell growth and death. Acta Neuropathol. 2012 May;123(5):711-25.

[68] Xie H, Wang M, Bonaldo Mde F, Rajaram V, Stellpflug W, Smith C, et al. Epigenomic analysis of Alu repeats in human ependymomas. Proc Natl Acad Sci U S A. 2010 Apr 13;107(15):6952-7.

Chapter 6

Carbonic Anhydrase IX in Adult and Pediatric Brain Tumors

Kristiina Nordfors, Joonas Haapasalo,
Hannu Haapasalo and Seppo Parkkila

Additional information is available at the end of the chapter

1. Introduction

Carbonic anhydrases (CAs) are zinc-containing metalloenzymes present in prokaryotes and eukaryotes (Sly and Hu 1995). CAs have been investigated since 1930's (Meldrum and Roughton 1933). They are important in normal human physiology, e.g., in gluconeogenesis, lipogenesis, ureagenesis, bone resorption, and formation of gastric juice and cerebrospinal fluid (Sly and Hu 1995, Pastoreková et al. 2004). There are at least 15 members in human alpha-CA family: Five active family members are cytosolic (CA I-III, VII, and XIII), four are membrane associated (CA IV, IX, XII, and XIV), two are mitochondrial (CA VA and VB), and one is a secretory form (CA VI). In addition, there are three acatalytic forms, which are called CA-related protein (CARPs). CAs can be categorized to catalytically active or inactive, intracellular or extracellular, and wide-spread or restricted to few tissues.

Their main physiological fuction is to catalyze the conversion of CO2 to bicarbonate ion and proton, as described by the following reaction:

$$CO_2 + H_2O \overset{CA}{\longleftrightarrow} HCO_3^- + H^+$$

In addition to their functions in normal physiology, the roles of CAs in different diseases have been extensively investigated during the last decades. They are involved in certain neurological and hereditary disorders, oedema, and most importantly, in cancer. There are at least three tumor associated isoforms; CA II, IX and XII. Especially carbonic anhydrase IX (CA IX) has been associated to neoplastic growth and cancer. The following chapter will discuss the role of CA IX in brain tumors.

2. Carbonic anhydrase IX

Carbonic anhydrase IX was first found by Pastroreková et al. (1992) and the *CA9* gene was cloned by the Pastrorek et al. (1994). Previously, a research group from Netherlands described a monoclonal antibody, named G250, which stained cell membranes of renal cell carcinoma, but did not stain normal epithelium (Oosterwijk et al. 1986). They continued their studies to establish G250 as a tool in cancer diagnostics and treatment. Afterwards, the protein recognized by the G250 antibody was characterized to be CA IX (Grabmaier et al. 2000).

CA 9 gene was originally located to the chromosome 17q21.2 by fluorescence in situ hybridization (Opavský et al. 1996), but it was later localized to the chromosome 9p13-p12 by radiation hybrid mapping (http://www.ncbi.nlm.nih.gov/gene/768). *CA9* gene consists of eleven exons and ten introns (Opavský et al. 1996), and encodes a protein containing 466 amino acids. It has a proteoglycan (PG) domain, central catalytic (CA) domain, transmembrane anchor, and short COOH- terminal cytoplasmic tail. CA IX was initially called MN, found from human carcinoma cell line, and later associated to neoplastic growth in carcinomas of ovary, uterine cervix and endometrium (Závada et al. 1993). A detailed characterisation of human CA IX protein has has shown that the recombinant CA IX protein exhibits the highest catalytic activity ever measured for any CA isozyme (Hilvo et al. 2008).

3. Carbonic anhydrase IX in normal tissue

The expression of CA IX in normal tissues has been thoroughly investigated. In mouse tissues, the highest expression has been detected in gastric mucosa, moderate expression in colon and brain, whereas low expression has been reported in pancreas and small intestine (Hilvo et al. 2004). The similar distribution pattern has been detected in human tissues; high CA IX staining has been discovered in GI-tract, especially in the epithelia of the gallbladder and gastric mucosa (Pastorek et al. 1994, Pastoreková et al. 1997, Saarnio et al. 1998a). Furthermore, Saarnio et al. (1998b) have reported the most intensive signals of CA IX in the epitelium of the duodenum and jejunum, whereas the expression diminishes towards the large intestine. Mesothelium, epithelial cells of the esophagus, and pancreatic and biliary ducts express CA IX (Turner et al. 1997, Pastoreková et al. 1997, Kivelä et al. 2000, Ivanov et al. 2001). CA IX has been detected in the male reproductive organs, whereas the female reproductive tract express only low amounts of CA IX (Liao et al. 1994; Karhumaa et al. 2001). Generally, expression of CA IX is generally low in the human brain, although positive signal has been reported in the epithelial cells of the choroid plexus (Ivanov et al. 2001, Proescholdt et al. 2005). Similarly, lower levels of CA IX mRNA have been reported in the normal brain as compared to brain neoplasms (Said et al. 2007a).

4. Carbonic anhydrase IX in neoplastic tissue

The von Hippel–Lindau (*VHL*) tumor suppressor gene was the first link to the major pathway controlling CA IX expression (Wykoff et al. 2000). Importantly, CA IX turned out to be one of the enzymes regulated by the hypoxia pathway, in which hypoxia inducible factor 1 (HIF-1) plays a role as a key transcription factor, especially in hypoxic tumors. Under normoxia, the encoded VHL protein (pVHL) binds to hydroxylated hypoxia inducible factor 1 – alpha and causes degradation by the ubiquitin-mediated proteasome system, inactivating the down-stream target genes. (Ivanov et al.1998). HIF-1 is stabilized under hypoxic conditions and binds to hypoxia-responsive elements in many genes, e.g VEGF, erythropoietin, and glucose transporter. This leads to the induction of erythropoiesis, angiogenesis, and glycolysis (Carmeliet et al. 1998). HIF-1 also activates *CA9* gene and CA IX expression level increases dramatically in hypoxic conditions. In line with this, high CA IX expression is often found in perinecrotic regions of tumors (Wykoff et al. 2000). The similar induction of CA IX has been proposed to take place in brain tumors. CA IX mRNA has been studied in human malignant glioma cell lines and distinct patterns of hypoxic expression of CA IX have been observed (Said et al. 2007b). The finding indicated that low oxygen concentration is probably the driving force for the increased CA IX expression due to the presence of a hypoxia responsive element (HRE) in the *CA9* promoter (Wykoff et al. 2000). The activation of hypoxia-inducible genes is illustrated in Figure 1.

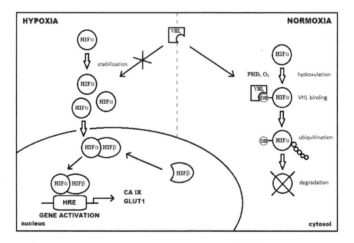

Figure 1. Activation of hypoxia-inducible genes. Under normoxia, HIFα is degraded by ubiquitin-proteasome system. Prolyl-4-hydroxylases (PHD) hydroxylate two conserved proline residues of HIF-1α, then von Hippel-Lindau protein (VHL) binds to the hydroxylated HIF-1α. Under hypoxia, PHDs are inactive in the absence of dioxygen, and HIF-1α is not recognized by VHL protein. HIF-1α accumulates and is translocated to the nucleus. HIF-1β constitutive subunit dimerizes with HIF-1α, resulting in the active transcription factor, which binds to hypoxia response element (HRE). Therefore the transcription of target genes, such as *CA9* and *GLUT1*, is induced. Adapted from Pastoreková et al. (2008) and Haapasalo (2011).

The overexpression of CAIX in majority of renal cell carcinomas (RCCs) is due to the loss of functional VHL protein, which causes the stabilization of HIF-1. (Gnarra et al. 1994, Wykoff et al. 2000). In other words, the CAs are no longer regulated by hypoxia. On the contrary, the majority of tumors do not contain VHL mutations, and in these, CA IX is usually found in focal perinecrotic areas, supporting the role of hypoxia in CA IX regulation (Wykoff et al. 2000). Furthermore, it has been suggested that HIF activates genes that change the expression profile of tumor cells suffering from hypoxia; thus, either leading to adaptation to the hypoxic stress or resulting in cell death. If this adaptation is successful, the surviving tumor cell population is associated with increasingly aggressive behaviour involving invasion and metastases, resistance to anti-cancer treatment, and finally, worse patient prognosis. (Harris 2002). This mechanism is supported by various immunohistochemical studies in which the CA IX expression is located in in the perinecrotic regions of solid tumors.

The mechanisms behind the role of CA IX in cancer have been studied widely. The hypoxia, measured by needle electrores, has been shown to correlate with CA IX expression in cervical cancer (Loncaster et al. 2001). This finding has been further clarified in genetic analysis, showing that *CA9* was the most induced gene among the 32 identified hypoxia responsive genes, which included *VEGF*, in human solid tumors (Lal et al. 2002). *In vitro*, *CA9* has been shown to be hypoxia-regulated in glioblastoma cells (Said et al. 2008).

The pivotal feature of the malignant tumor cells is their capability to maintain the normal intracellular pH, whereas the extracellular pH is significantly acidic. CA IX increases the extracellular acidification by shifting the site of CO_2 hydration from intra- to extracellular (Svastová et al. 2004). This in turn increases the capability of tumor cells to survive and invade, and the selective sulfonamide inhibitors disturb this process. Acetazolamide, a potent CA inhibitor, has been shown to suppress the invasion of renal cancer cells *in vitro* (Parkkila et al. 2000b). Interestingly, CA IX has an optimal catalytic activity for CO_2 hydration to bicarbonate and proton in acidic pH (Innocenti et al. 2009). Furthermore, when studied in cancer-derived cell lines, CA IX diminishes the intracellular pH gradient in the hypoxic core of three-dimensional tumor spheroids (Swietach et al. 2008). These findings support the theory that CA IX is an essential factor for tumor cells in adaptation to hypoxia and their survival, and is illustared in Figure 2.

Even though the expression of CA IX is mainly regulated by hypoxia, it has been shown that acidosis increases CA IX expression via a hypoxia-independent mechanism (Ihnatko et al. 2006). CA IX has been proposed to be regulated by low oxygen concentrations or constitutive, oncogene-related mechanisms (Said et al. 2007a). Furthermore, CA IX modulates E-cadherin mediated cell adhesion by decreasing the binding of this cell adhesion molecule to beta-catenin (Svastová et al. 2003). This, in turn, could possibly benefit the cancer cells by an increase in cell motility and invasion. As mentioned before, acetazolamide can suppress the invasion of renal cancer cells *in vitro* (Parkkila et al. 2000b). However, the inhibition of CA IX in RNAi-treated breast cancer cells reduced the invasion capacity only slightly (Robertson et al. 2004). There is also evidence that CA IX expression is a negative predictive factor when evaluating the treatment efficacy in oestrogen receptor-positive tumors treated with adjuvant tamoxifen after

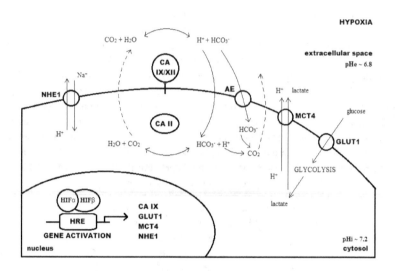

Figure 2. Example of pH regulation in a cancer cell under hypoxia. This is controlled by HIF-1 mediated gene activation. The rapid metabolic rate requires glucose which is transported to the cell by the glucose transporter (GLUT1). Glycolysis produces lactate and protons, which are transported to extracellular space by the H^+/monocarboxylate transporter 4 (MCT4). The transmebrane CA IX (and XII), and cytosolic CA II prevent intracellular acidification and maintain the physiological pH. Anion exchangers (AE) transport bicarbonate to cytosol, which then buffers the protons produced by the active metabolism. Resulting CO_2 is secreted from the cell by diffusion. The Na^+/H^+ exchanger 1 (NHE1) participates in the secretion of proton. The HIF-mediated machinery and oncogenic pathways result in secretion of protons and CO_2 to extracellular space, thus promoting the breakdown of the extracellular matrix and invasion of tumor cells. Adapted from Pastoreková et al. (2008) and Haapasalo (2011).

primary chemo-endocrine therapy (Generali et al. 2006). The role of CA IX in resistance to chemotherapy could be explained by the effects of pH on tamoxifen uptake.

Ectopic expression of CA IX is induced in various tumors. These include the malignancies of breast, cervix uteri, esophagus, kidney, and lung (Liao et al. 1994, McKiernan et al. 1997, Liao et al. 1997, Turner et al. 1997, Vermylen et al. 1999, Bartosová et al. 2002). When these tumors are considered, CA IX is absent in the corresponding normal tissue. Conversely, CA IX expression is usually absent or reduced in tumors which have originated from CA IX-positive tissues. These include carcinomas of stomach and gallbladder (Saarnio et al. 2001, Leppilampi et al. 2003). This makes the CA IX a promising molecule as a prognostic factor as well as a potential target for therapeutic methods.

In cervical cancer, the CA IX expression correlates to tumor hypoxia and poor patient prognosis, and could be used in the selection of suitable patients for hypoxia-modification therapies (Loncaster et al. 2001). In lung cancer CA IX is a marker of poor prognosis (Swinson et al. 2003, Kim et al. 2004), and it has been associated to proteins linked to angiogenesis, disruption of cell-cell adhesion and inhibition of apoptosis (Giatromanolaki et al. 2001). CA IX could also been used as a differentiation tool between preneoplastic lesions and lung cancer (Vermylen et al. 1998) and a high concentration of CA IX in plasma serves as a independent prognostic biomarker in patients with non-small cell lung cancer (Ilie et al. 2010). CA IX expression is sensitive for diagnostics of mesothelioma and metastatic clear cell renal cell carcinoma of the lung (Ramsey et al. 2012). Furthermore, CA IX expression has been associated with poor prognosis for patients with head and neck cancer (Beasley et al. 2001, Koukourakis et al. 2001), esophageal cancer (Birner et al. 2011), ovarian cancer (Hynninen et al. 2006, Choschzick et al. 2011), soft tissue sarcoma (Måseide et al. 2004), and bladder carcinoma (Hoskin et al. 2003). It has been confirmed in several studies that CA IX correlates with poor prognosis in breast cancer (Chia et al. 2001, Brennan et al. 2006, Hussain et al. 2007) and is related to overexpression of c-erbB2 (Bartosová et al. 2002).

The most widely investigated tumor type, considering CA IX, is renal cell carcinoma (RCC) in which CA IX represents a useful marker (Liao et al. 1997, McKiernan et al. 1997, Parkkila et al. 2000a). In its most common subtype, clear cell carcinoma, CA IX expression is higher than in other renal cell cancer types (Sandlund et al. 2007). In addition, patients with both conventional renal cell cancer and low CA IX expression had a less favourable prognosis. In renal cancer CA IX is a promising therapeutic target for novel oncological applications, including immunotherapy and radioisotopic methods (Pastoreková et al. 2006, Bleumer et al. 2006). CA IX and CA XII are functionally involved in tumor growth (Chiche et al. 2009). Renal cell cancer *in vivo* experiments showed that *CA9* gene silencing alone led to a 40% reduction in xenograft tumor volume, and silencing of both *CA9* and *CA12* resulted in an 85% reduction in tumor volume.

5. Carbonic anhydrases in adult brain tumors

The incidence of brain tumors is similar in different countries and rather stable over the past two decades (Pollack et al. 2011). There are about 50 new pediatric and 1000 adult brain tumors every year in Finland with five million habitants (Statistics Finland 2011). The etiology of brain tumors has been under intense investigation but no clear evidence between different environmental, nutritional or lifestyle and carcinogenesis have been found (Baldwin et al. 2004). Most common primary CNS tumors of the adult are gliomas and meningiomas. Glioblastoma is a highly malignant and unfortunately common, glial tumor and the 5-year survival of the patients is less than 10 % (Stupp et al. 2009). On the other hand, almost all (90-98%) patients with meningioma are alive after five years (Statistics Finland 2011).

The expression of carbonic anhydrases in brain tumors has been previously reported (Parkkila AK et al. 1995). The first findings assessed CA II, which was stained positively by immunohistochemistry in astrocytic tumors, oligodendrogliomas and medulloblastomas. The expression of CA IX was first reported by Ivanov et. al (2001). In this first study, they screened tumors of different genetic background as well as several malignant cell lines for the expression of CA IX. mRNA analysis revealed high-to-moderate levels of expression of *CA9* and *CA12* in glioma cell lines. Immunolocalization of CA IX was further studied in 11 gliomas; low-grade gliomas were not stained for CA IX, whereas grade III-IV gliomas were all CA IX positive. In addition, 3 oligodendrogliomas were included in the analysis and they failed to express CA IX. Furthermore, all hemangioblastomas (3 tumors), meningiomas (5 tumors), and two out of three choroid plexus tumors were positive for CA IX.

This overview of different tumors was followed by a study of Proescholdt et al. (2005) on CA IX and CA XII, which combined brain tumors of different histology and grade of malignancy. The material consisted of total of 112 tumor samples (grade I-IV astrocytomas, meningiomas, metastases, primitive neuroectodermal tumors (PNETs), and hemangioblastomas). Generally, low-grade astrocytomas did not show any positive staining for CA IX and the expression increased with increasing WHO grade. The strongest staining of all glioma samples was observed in the glioblastomas, and almost all of the samples (97%) were positive. In these, the staining was detected around necrotic areas. However, more diffuse staining pattern without any association to necrosis was detected and CA IX expression was found in almost all tumor cells, including those near blood vessels, suggesting the induction also without the hypoxia-inducible mechanism. In the meningiomas, increased CA IX staining, with diffuse and evenly distributed pattern, was found in comparison to the normal brain. The authors found the most widespread CA IX and XII staining of all tumors in hemangioblastoma samples.

As to brain tumors, the first large study to describe the expression of CA IX in human diffusely infiltrating astrocytomas was published year after (Haapasalo et al. 2006). The study material consisted of 362 diffusely infiltrating astrocytoma samples (grades II-IV), which were obtained from surgically operated patients. Cellular CA IX immunopositivity was observed in 78% of diffusely infiltrating astrocytomas and the percentages according the WHO grade were as follows; 65% of grade II astrocytomas, 73% of grade 3 astrocytomas, and 82% of grade 4 astrocytomas. The immunohistochemial results were verified by mRNA analysis. The statistical comparison of cytoplasmic CA IX intensity and tumor grade revealed significantly higher CA IX intensity in tumors of higher malignancy grade. Again, CA IX was expressed in areas close to the necrotic regions and cytoplasmic staining was seen in the neoplastic cells of the infiltrative zone. When important clinicopathologial features were assessed, CA IX showed no association with p53 expression nor did it correlate with epidermal growth factor receptor–amplification, apoptosis, or cell proliferation by Ki-67/MIB-1. There was a significant correlation between increasing CA IX intensity and increasing patient age. For the first time, CA IX positivity was associated to shortened patient survival in univariate analysis: CA IX intensity divided the tumors into four significantly differing prognostic subsets (Figure 3). The survival difference was even significant within grade II and grade IV tumors separately. Most importantly, statistical analysis of the data revealed that the patient age, tumor grade, and CA IX intensity all had independent prognostic value when evaluated by Cox multivariate analysis.

The finding that CA IX predicts poor prognosis has been confirmed by others. Korkolopoulou et al. (2007) showed that increasing CA IX immunopositivity was associated with a shortened survival in univariate analysis. Furthermore, they reported similar independent prognosticators in multivariate analysis including CA IX, tumor grade and patient age. The perinecrotic distribution of CA IX immunostaining was detected and intensity increased in parallel with the extent of necrosis and histological grade. In concordance, Sathornsumetee et al. (2008) conducted a trial, in which patients with recurrent malignant astrocytomas treated with a combination of VEGF -neutralizing antibodies were retrospectively evaluated. Survival

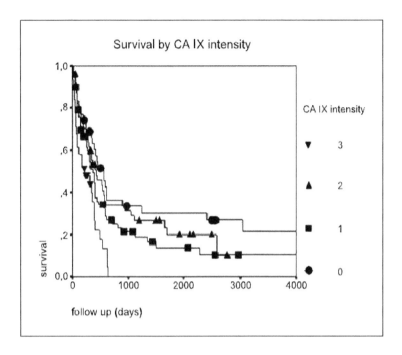

Figure 3. Prognostic significance of CA IX in diffusely infiltrating astrocytomas (grades II-IV). Kaplan-Meier curves are shown (p = 0.0011, log-rank test). Haapasalo J et al. (2006)

analysis revealed that high CA IX expression was associated with poor survival outcome. VEGF was associated with radiographic response but not with survival. Interestingly, they tested both CA IX and HIF simultaneously in a Cox model as separate factors, and only CA IX remained as a statistically significant factor. One opposite result has been published in glioma patient cohort (Flynn et al. 2008). In this study, no significant correlations between the CA IX expression and patient survival or tumor grade were found, although the patients with CA IX-positive tumors seemed to have a trend towards a worse prognosis. This might be due to different immunostaining method used. The most reliable method for CA IX immunostaining having no cross-reactivity with other CAs (Saarnio et al. 1998b), is based on M75 antibodies used by us and e.g. Korkolopoulou et al. (2007). Flynn et al. (2008) had also smaller number of patients. Yoo et. al (2010) assessed the issue again, and showed that CA IX expression was a predictive factor for poor survival and correlated positively with increasing WHO grade.

The expression of CA IX has been studied in other gliomas as well. Järvelä et al. (2008) showed by immunohistochemistry that 80% of studied 86 oligodendroglial tumors stained positively for CA IX. In addition, CA IX predicted poor prognosis in univariate analysis and in multivariate analysis CA IX expression, patient age and histological component (pure oligodendroglioma vs. mixed oligoastrocytoma) showed independent prognostic values. Abraham et al. (2012) have recently assessed the expression of all hypoxia related molecules HIF-1, VEGF, Glut-1, and CA IX, in oligodendrogliomas. They found that all these proteins were statistically significantly different between grade II and III oligodendrogliomas, anaplastic oligodendrogliomas having stronger expression. Ingterestingly, low CA IX expression predicted better prognosis in anaplastic oligodendrogliomas but not in grade II oligodendrogliomas, whereas the prognostic significance was not reported in the whole tumor material.

As for mostly benign tumors, Yoo et al. (2007) showed that 50% of all meningiomas contained regions of hypoxia as judged by expression of CA IX. CA IX expression was significantly associated with higher-grade histology and tended to be more common in recurrent tumors. Futhermore, Korhonen et al. (2009) reported 11.6% cytosolic CA IX expression in meningiomas. CA IX positivity was neither associated with the studied clinicopathological factors nor survival.

Recently, Jensen et al. (2012) assessed the molecular markers of hypoxia, vascularity, and proliferation in meningeomas, including CA IX. As expected, VEGF, HIF, CA IX, and Glut-1 were positively correlated. There was an association between higher-grade tumors with higher scores for CA IX, VEGF, and HIF-1alpha, but CA IX was not associated to overall survival.

CA IX is also significantly upregulated in craniopharyngiomas and is associated with increased cyst size (Proescholdt et al. 2011). The mechanisms of CA IX regulation remain unknown, since neither hypoxia nor p53 appear to play a role in these tumors. The authors state, that inhibition of CA IX may be a potential target for the adjuvant treatment in patients with cystic craniopharyngiomas.

6. CA IX in pediatric brain tumors

Pediatric cancers are still the main cause of death in children aged 1-14 years in the UK and Finland (Gatta et al. 2005, Statistics Finland 2011). After leukemia brain tumors are the second most common tumor group. Approximately 60-70% of the patients with brain tumors are alive five years from the diagnosis (Pokhrel and Hakulinen 2009). The most common pediatric brain tumors are pilocytic astrosytoma, medulloblastoma and ependymoma. Neurosurgical operation is the most important treatment modality. Inoperable or highly malignant tumors are treated also with radio- and chemotherapy. CNS is vulnerable, especially when evolving. Most of the patients do survive but the tumor and the different treatment modalities can cause side effects that reduce the quality of life. Supratentorial tumors, tumor reoperations, shunt revisions and chemotherapy increase the risk of these problems (Reimers et al. 2003, Pietilä et al. 2012). There is only a limited scope for improvement with conventional chemotherapy and thus, there is an urgent need of therapeutic agents for these patients. CA IX is one novel molecule that might serve as a prognostic/diagnostic tool, and perhaps, a target for various therapeutic methods.

Some publications have assessed the CA IX expression in pediatric brain tumors. Ivanov et al. (2001) screened a small amount of brain tumors and found the following inmmunohistochemistry results: most of the 7 central/peripheral PNETs expressed the CA IX, all of 6 studied epedymomas were posivive. Preusser et al. (2005) assessed the CA IX in intracranial ependy-momas: 84 out of 100 tumors expressed CA IX, and it was associated with a bizarre angiogen-esis and necrosis. However, CA IX failed to reach a prognostic significance in univariate analysis. The most common, solid, extracranial pediatric nervous tumor is neuroblastoma. Dungwa et al. (2012) found positive membranous/cytoplasmic CA IX expression in 21 (23%) of 91 neuroblastomas but was absent in ganglioneuromas. Neuroblastomas with 1p deletion and MYCN amplification had even stronger membranous expression. 18% of the neuroblas-tomas showed nuclear CA IX expression in 10% or more tumoral cells. Nuclear CA IX expression associated with worse overall –and event-free survival.

We have previously studied CA IX in 39 medulloblastomas and PNETs (Nordfors et al. 2010). CA IX positivity was found in 23% of tumors and the expression was linked to necrosis. CA IX expression was analysed in concordance with various clinical features and molecular markers. Proliferation (Ki-67/MIB-1), apoptosis or expression of Bcl-2, p53 or c-erbB-2 were not associated with CA IX in any of the groups except for the correlation between positive c-erbB-2 and positive CA IX expression in PNETs. CA IX was also positively associated with female gender. There was no significant difference in the expression of CA IX between primary and recurrent tumors in any of the groups. Moreover, there was no correlation between the tumor type (MBs/PNETs) and CA IX intensity. Interestingly, CA IX-positivity was a marker of worse outcome in patients with MB/PNET in univariate and multivariate analyses (Figure 4). Generally, CA IX is associated with higher grade, necrosis, and worse CA IX seems to have several inductors. CA IX is often found in perinecrotic areas. Because necrosis is an uncommon feature and is not considered to be a significant prognostic factor in MBs, the induction of CA IX in MBs/PNETs may also involve hypoxia-independent mechanisms. In addition, there is the evidence that CA IX is expressed in grade I pilocytic astrocytomas, and the immunoposi-tivity for CA IX is associated to histopathological features of degeneration and increased proliferation (our unpublished results).

In children, possible side-effects of therapeutic interventions may be more severe and the exact biology of hypoxia and its clinical relevance in childhood tumors is still unclear. Thus, further studies will be needed before novel agents concerning hypoxia can be introduced into pediatric oncology.

7. Future aspects

The tumor tissue specific CA IX expression has led researchers to propose several novel treatment strategies. A promising treatment strategy is to use CA selective inhibitors (Pastoreková et al. 2004). Tumor cells probably use CAs as key enzymes to adapt to the hostile environment caused by metabolic stress of cancer cells, and thus, acidification facilitates the spread and invasion of cancer cells (Svastová et al. 2004). High CA IX expression might increase the capability of cells to infiltrate the neighboring tissue. The inhibition of this process would potentially disturb the invasion processes of cancer cells.

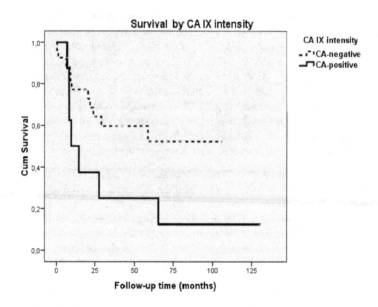

Figure 4. Prognostic significance of CA IX in medulloblastomas/PNETs. Kaplan-Meier curves are shown (P = 0.041, log-rank test). Nordfors et al. (2010)

Another possible treatment option is to use cancer-specific antibodies. The CA and proteo-glycan domains give the molecule a unique extracellular structure. CA IX expression is high in renal cell carcinoma (Liao et al. 1997) and this has enabled therapeutic trials with high-dose radiolabeled CA IX antibody (cG250) and CA IX-loaded dendritic cells. Unfortunately, a significant breakthrough in clinical trials remains to be achieved and in RCC trials are still in phase II (Stillebroer et al. 2010).

CA IX could also be used as a potential target for immune therapy. Greiner et al. (2006) found a significant correlation between high mRNA levels of CA IX and a longer overall survival in acute myeloid leukemia. This might be due to the induction of a strong antileukemic immune response by CA IX. Similar findings have been found in metastatic RCC patients (Uemura et al. 2006). Vaccination with tumor-RNA pulsed dendritic cells led to increased numbers of CA IX peptide-specific cytotoxic T76 lymphocytes and IgG levels without any major adverse event. Metastasis of three patients shrank or even disappeared and the overall survival was longer for six patients. However, further studies are required to confirm these findings in larger study cohorts.

Bevacizumab, an anti-VEGF antibody, inhibits the developing vasculature of tumors, but resistance is common. Antiangiogenic therapy induces hypoxia and thus, CA IX. Curious-ly, McIntyre et al. (2012) knocked down CAIX expression in a colon cancer and a glioblas-toma cell lines and combined the results with bevacizumab. They found that CAIX expression was associated with increased necrosis and apoptosis *in vivo* and *in vitro*. Added to this, acidity seemed to inhibit CAIX activity, and this may be the mechanism whereby excess acid self-limits the build-up of extracellular acid. It seems that inhibition of the hypoxic adaptation to antiangiogenic therapy enhances bevacizumab treatment and highlights the value of developing small molecules or antibodies which inhibit CAIX for combination therapy.

8. Conclusions

CA IX has been linked to several cancer tissues, whereas the normal tissue is mostly negative. This seems to be the case also when different brain tumors are concerned. Malignant astrocytomas and oligodendrogliomas express CA IX and it has been shown as a useful prognosticator. Being a hypoxia/necrosis marker, CA IX can be used as a diagnostic tool in the grading of astrocytomas and oligodendrogliomas. Tumor biopsies containing a small amount of tissue for diagnosis, are especially good targets. In addition, CA IX is associated to more malignant phenotype in meningiomas and some other mostly benign brain tumors.

CA IX is present in the most common malignant brain tumor of children, medulloblastoma, as well as in PNETs. Interestingly, in these tumors CA IX predicts poor prognosis and could be used as a marker when planning the cancer therapy. Added to this, CA IX has been shown to be expressed in other pediatric brain tumors, such as ependymomas and pilocytic astrocytomas, where it is linked to degenerative histopathological features.

CA IX is associated with hypoxia, necrosis, and angiogenesis – features traditionally linked to the tumorigenesis of brain tumors. Several studies show that CA IX could be used as a target molecule in adult and pediatric brain tumors. Further clinical trials for cancer treatment are needed aiming to either eradicate the tumor cell population or turn the tumor into a more chronic and stable disease.

Author details

Kristiina Nordfors[1], Joonas Haapasalo[2], Hannu Haapasalo[3] and Seppo Parkkila[4]

1 Department of Pediatrics, Tampere University Hospital, Tampere, Finland

2 Unit of Neurosurgery, Tampere University Hospital, Tampere, Finland

3 Department of Pathology, Fimlab Ltd and Tampere University Hospital, Tampere, Finland

4 Department of Anatomy, Tampere University, Fimlab Ltd and Tampere University Hospital, Tampere, Finland

References

[1] Abraham S, Hu N, Jensen R (2012); Hypoxia-inducible factor-1-regulated protein ex-
     pression and oligodendroglioma patient outcome: comparison with established bio-
     markers and preoperative UCSF low-grade scoring system. J Neurooncol. 108:459-68.

[2] Baldwin RT, Preston-Martin S (2004); Epidemiology of brain tumors in childhood – a
     review. Toxicol Appl Pharmacol 199:118-31.

[3] Bartosová M, Parkkila S, Pohlodek K, Karttunen TJ, Galbavý S, Mucha V, Harris AL,
     Pastorek J, Pastoreková S (2002); Expression of carbonic anhydrase IX in breast is as-
     sociated with malignant tissues and is related to overexpression of c-erbB2. J. Pathol.
     197:314-21.

[4] Beasley NJ, Wykoff CC, Watson PH, Leek R, Turley H, Gatter K, Pastorek J, Cox GJ,
     Ratcliffe P, Harris AL (2001); Carbonic anhydrase IX, an endogenous hypoxia mark-
     er, expression in head and neck squamous cell carcinoma and its relationship to hy-
     poxia, necrosis, and microvessel density. Cancer Res. 61:5262-7.

[5] Birner P, Jesch B, Friedrich J, Riegler M, Zacherl J, Hejna M, Wrba F, Schultheis A,
     Schoppmann SF (2011); Carbonic Anhydrase IX Overexpression is Associated with
     Diminished Prognosis in Esophageal Cancer and Correlates with Her-2 Expression;
     Ann. Surg. Oncol. 18:3330-7.

[6] Bleumer I, Oosterwijk E, Oosterwijk-Wakka JC, Völler MC, Melchior S, Warnaar SO,
     Mala C, Beck J, Mulders PF (2006); A clinical trial with chimeric monoclonal antibody
     WX-G250 and low dose interleukin-2 pulsing scheme for advanced renal cell carcino-
     ma. J. Urol. 175:57-62.

[7] Brennan DJ, Jirstrom K, Kronblad A, Millikan RC, Landberg G, Duffy MJ, Rydén L,
     Gallagher WM, O'Brien SL (2006); CA IX is an independent prognostic marker in pre-
     menopausal breast cancer patients with one to three positive lymph nodes and a pu-
     tative marker of radiation resistance. Clin. Cancer Res. 12:6421-31.

[8] Carmeliet P, Dor Y, Herbert JM, Fukumura D, Brusselmans K, Dewerchin M, Nee-
     man M, Bono F, Abramovitch R, Maxwell P, Koch CJ, Ratcliffe P, Moons L, Jain RK,
     Collen D, Keshert E, Keshet E (1998); Role of HIF-1alpha in hypoxia-mediated apop-
     tosis, cell proliferation and tumour angiogenesis. Nature 394:485-490.

[9] Chia SK, Wykoff CC, Watson PH, Han C, Leek RD, Pastorek J, Gatter KC, Ratcliffe P,
     Harris AL (2001); Prognostic significance of a novel hypoxia-regulated marker, car-
     bonic anhydrase IX, in invasive breast carcinoma. J. Clin. Oncol. 19:3660-8.

[10] Chiche J, Ilc K, Laferrière J, Trottier E, Dayan F, Mazure NM, Brahimi-Horn MC,
     Pouysségur J (2009); Hypoxia-inducible carbonic anhydrase IX and XII promote tu-
     mour cell growth by counteracting acidosis through the regulation of the intracellu-
     lar pH. Cancer Res. 69:358-68.

[11] Choschzick M, Oosterwijk E, Müller V, Woelber L, Simon R, Moch H, Tennstedt P (2011); Overexpression of carbonic anhydrase IX (CAIX) is an independent unfavorable prognostic marker in endometrioid ovarian cancer. Virchows Arch. 459:193-200.

[12] Dungwa JV, Hunt LP, Ramani P (2012); Carbonic anhydrase IX up-regulation is associated with adverse clinicopathologic and biologic factors in neuroblastomas. Hum Pathol. 43:1651-60.

[13] Flynn JR, Wang L, Gillespie DL, Stoddard GJ, Reid JK, Owens J, Ellsworth GB, Salzman KL, Kinney AY, Jensen RL (2008); Hypoxia-regulated protein expression, patient characteristics, and preoperative imaging as predictors of survival in adults with glioblastoma multiforme. Cancer 113:1032-42.

[14] Gatta G, Capocaccia R, Stiller C, Kaatsch P, Berrino F and Terenziani M; EUROCARE Working Group (2005); Childhood cancer survival trends in Europe: a EUROCARE Working Group study. J Clin Oncol 23:3742-3751.

[15] Generali D, Fox SB, Berruti A, Brizzi MP, Campo L, Bonardi S, Wigfield SM, Bruzzi P, Bersiga A, Allevi G, Milani M, Aguggini S, Dogliotti L, Bottini A, Harris AL (2006); Role of carbonic anhydrase IX expression in prediction of the efficacy and outcome of primary epirubicin/tamoxifen therapy for breast cancer. Endocr. Relat. Cancer 13:921-30.

[16] Giatromanolaki A, Kukourakis MI, Sivridis E, Pastorek J, Wykoff CC, Gatter KC, Harris AL (2001); Expression of hypoxia-inducible carbonic anhydrase-9 relates to angiogenic pathways and independently to poor outcome in non-small cell lung cancer. Cancer Res. 61:7992-8.

[17] Gnarra JR, Tory K, Weng Y, Schmidt L, Wei MH, Li H, Latif F, Liu S, Chen F, Duh FM, et al. (1994); Mutations of the VHL tumour suppressor gene in renal carcinoma. Nat Genet. 7:85-90.

[18] Grabmaier K, Vissers JL, De Weijert MC, Oosterwijk-Wakka JC, Van Bokhoven A, Brakenhoff RH, Noessner E, Mulders PA, Merkx G, Figdor CG, Adema GJ, Oosterwijk E (2000); Molecular cloning and immunogenicity of renal cell carcinoma-associated antigen G250. Int J Cancer. 85:865-70.

[19] Haapasalo J (2011); Carbonic Anhydrases II, IX and XII in Astrocytic Gliomas: Their relationship with clinicopathological features and proliferation. PhD thesis. Acta Universitatis Tamperensis; 1647, Tampere University Press, Tampere.

[20] Haapasalo JA, Nordfors KM, Hilvo M, Rantala IJ, Soini Y, Parkkila AK, Pastoreková S, Pastorek J, Parkkila SM, Haapasalo HK (2006); Expression of carbonic anhydrase IX in astrocytic tumours predicts poor prognosis. Clin Cancer Res. 12:473-7.

[21] Harris AL (2002); Hypoxia–a key regulatory factor in tumour growth. Nature Rev. Cancer. 2: 38–47.

[22] Hilvo M, Baranauskiene L, Salzano AM, Scaloni A, Matulis D, Innocenti A, Scozzafava A, Monti SM, Di Fiore A, De Simone G, Lindfors M, Jänis J, Valjakka J, Pastoreko-

vá S, Pastorek J, Kulomaa MS, Nordlund HR, Supuran CT, Parkkila S. (2008); Biochemical characterization of CA IX: one of the most active carbonic anhydrase isozymes. J. Biol. Chem. 283:27799-809.

[23] Hoskin PJ, Sibtain A, Daley FM and Wilson GD (2003); GLUT1 and CAIX as intrinsic markers of hypoxia in bladder cancer: relationship with vascularity and proliferation as predictors of outcome of ARCON. J Cancer 89:1290-1297.

[24] Hussain SA, Ganesan R, Reynolds G, Gross L, Stevens A, Pastorek J, Murray PG, Perunovic B, Anwar MS, Billingham L, James ND, Spooner D, Poole CJ, Rea DW, Palmer DH (2007); Hypoxia-regulated carbonic anhydrase IX expression is associated with poor survival in patients with invasive breast cancer. Br. J. Cancer 96:104-9.

[25] Hynninen P, Vaskivuo L, Saarnio J, Haapasalo H, Kivelä J, Pastoreková S, Pastorek J, Waheed A, Sly WS, Puistola U, Parkkila S (2006); Expression of transmembrane carbonic anhydrases IX and XII in ovarian tumors. Histopathology 49:594-602.

[26] Ihnatko R, Kubes M, Takacova M, Sedlakova O, Sedlak J, Pastorek J, Kopacek J, Pastoreková S (2006); Extracellular acidosis elevates carbonic anhydrase IX in human glioblastoma cells via transcriptional modulation that does not depend on hypoxia. Int. J. Oncol. 29:1025-33.

[27] Ilie M, Mazure NM, Hofman V, Ammadi RE, Ortholan C, Bonnetaud C, Havet K, Venissac N, Mograbi B, Mouroux J, Pouysségur J, Hofman P (2010); High levels of carbonic anhydrase IX in tumour tissue and plasma are biomarkers of poor prognostic in patients with non-small cell lung cancer. Br J Cancer. 102:1627-35.

[28] Innocenti A, Pastoreková S, Pastorek J, Scozzafava A, De Simone G, Supuran CT (2009); The proteoglycan region of the tumor-associated carbonic anhydrase isoform IX acts as anintrinsic buffer optimizing CO2 hydration at acidic pH values characteristic of solid tumors. Bioorg Med Chem Lett. 19:5825-8.

[29] Ivanov SV, Kuzmin I, Wei M-H, Pack S, Geil L, Johnson BE, Stanbridge EJ, Lerman MI (1998); Down-regulation of transmembrane carbonic anhydrases in renal cell carcinoma cell lines by wild-type von Hippel-Lindau transgenes. Proc Natl Acad Sci USA 95:12596-12601.

[30] Ivanov S, Liao SY, Ivanova A, Danilkovitch-Miagkova A, Tarasova N, Weirich G, Merrill MJ, Proescholdt MA, Oldfield EH, Lee J, Zavada J, Waheed A, Sly W, Lerman MI and Stanbridge EJ (2001); Expression of hypoxia-inducible cell-surface transmembrane carbonic anhydrases in human cancer. Am J Pathol 158:905-919.

[31] Jensen R, Lee J (2012); Predicting outcomes of patients with intracranial meningiomas using molecular markers of hypoxia, vascularity, and proliferation. Neurosurgery. 71:146-56.

[32] Järvelä S, Parkkila S, Bragge H, Kähkönen M, Parkkila AK, Soini Y, Pastorekova S, Pastorek J, Haapasalo H (2008); Carbonic anhydrase IX in oligodendroglial brain tumors. BMC Cancer. 4;8:1.

[33] Karhumaa P, Kaunisto K, Parkkila S, Waheed A, Pastoreková S, Pastorek J, Sly WS, Rajaniemi H (2001); Expression of the transmembrane carbonic anhydrases, CA IX and CA XII, in the human male excurrent ducts. Mol Hum Reprod. 7:611-6.

[34] Kim SJ, Rabbani ZN, Vollmer RT, Schreiber EG, Oosterwijk E, Dewhirst MW, Vujaskovic Z, Kelley MJ (2004); Carbonic anhydrase IX in early-stage non-small cell lung cancer. Clin. Cancer Res. 10:7925-33.

[35] Kivelä AJ, Parkkila S, Saarnio J, Karttunen TJ, Kivelä J, Parkkila A-K, Pastoreková S, Pastorek J, Waheed A, Sly WS, Rajaniemi H (2000); Expression of transmembrane carbonic anhydrase isoenzymes IX and XII in normal human pancreas and pancreatic tumours. Histochem. Cell Biol. 114: 197-204.

[36] Korhonen K, Parkkila AK, Hélen P, Välimäki R, Pastoreková S, Pastorek J, Parkkila S, Haapasalo H (2009); Carbonic anhydrases in meningiomas: association of endothelial carbonic anhydrase II with aggressive tumor features. J Neurosurg. 111:472-7.

[37] Korkolopoulou P, Perdiki M, Thymara I, Boviatsis E, Agrogiannis G, Kotsiakis X, Angelidakis D, Rologis D, Diamantopoulou K, Thomas-Tsagli E, Kaklamanis L, Gatter K, Patsouris E (2007); Expression of hypoxia-related tissue factors in astrocytic gliomas. A multivariate survival study with emphasis upon carbonic anhydrase IX. Hum. Pathol. 38:629-38.

[38] Koukourakis MI, Giatromanolaki A, Sivridis E, Simopoulos K, Pastorek J, Wykoff CC, Gatter KC and Harris AL (2001); Hypoxia-regulated carbonic anhydrase-9 (CA9) relates to poor vascularization and resistance of squamous cell head and neck cancer to chemoradiotherapy. Clin Cancer Res 7:3399-3403.

[39] Lal A, Peters H, St Croix B, Haroon ZA, Dewhirst MW, Strausberg RL, Kaanders JH, van der Kogel AJ, Riggins GJ (2001); Transcriptional response to hypoxia in human tumors. J Natl Cancer Inst. 93:1337-43.

[40] Liao SY, Brewer C, Závada J, Pastorek J, Pastoreková S, Manetta A, Berman ML, DiSaia PJ, Stanbridge EJ (1994); Identification of the MN antigen as a diagnostic biomarker of cervical intraepithelial squamous and glandular neoplasia and cervical carcinomas. Am. J. Pathol. 145:598-609.

[41] Liao SY, Aurelio ON, Jan K, Zavada J, Stanbridge EJ (1997); Identification of the MN/CA9 protein as a reliable diagnostic biomarker of clear cell carcinoma of the kidney. Cancer Res 57:2827-31.

[42] Loncaster JA, Harris AL, Davidson SE, Logue JP, Hunter RD, Wycoff CC, Pastorek J, Ratcliffe PJ, Stratford IJ, West CM (2001); Carbonic anhydrase (CA IX) expression, a potential new intrinsic marker of hypoxia: correlations with tumor oxygen measure-

ments and prognosis in locally advanced carcinoma of the cervix. Cancer Res. 61:6394-9.

[43] Liao SY, Brewer C, Závada J, Pastorek J, Pastoreková S, Manetta A, Berman ML, DiSaia PJ, Stanbridge EJ (1994); Identification of the MN antigen as a diagnostic biomarker of cervical intraepithelial squamous and glandular neoplasia and cervical carcinomas. Am. J. Pathol. 145:598-609.

[44] Liao SY, Aurelio ON, Jan K, Zavada J, Stanbridge EJ (1997); Identification of the MN/CA9 protein as a reliable diagnostic biomarker of clear cell carcinoma of the kidney. Cancer Res 57:2827-31.

[45] Loncaster JA, Harris AL, Davidson SE, Logue JP, Hunter RD, Wycoff CC, Pastorek J, Ratcliffe PJ, Stratford IJ, West CM (2001); Carbonic anhydrase (CA IX) expression, a potential new intrinsic marker of hypoxia: correlations with tumor oxygen measurements and prognosis in locally advanced carcinoma of the cervix. Cancer Res. 61:6394-9.

[46] McIntyre A, Patiar S, Wigfield S, Li JL, Ledaki I, Turley H, Leek R, Snell C, Gatter K, Sly WS, Vaughan-Jones RD, Swietach P, Harris AL. Carbonic Anhydrase IX Promotes Tumor Growth and Necrosis In Vivo and Inhibition Enhances Anti-VEGF Therapy (2012); Clin Cancer Res. 18:3100-11.

[47] McKiernan JM, Buttyan R, Bander NH, Stifelman MD, Katz AE, Chen MW, Olsson CA, Sawczuk IS (1997); Expression of the tumor-associated gene MN: a potential biomarker for human renal cell carcinoma. Cancer Res. 57:2362-5.

[48] Meldrum NU and Roughton FJW (1933); Carbonic anhydrase. Its preparation and properties. J Physiol (London) 80:113-142.

[49] Måseide K, Kandel RA, Bell RS, Catton CN, O'Sullivan B, Wunder JS, Pintilie M, Hedley D, Hill RP (2004); Carbonic anhydrase IX as a marker for poor prognosis in soft tissue sarcoma. Clin. Cancer Res. 10:4464-71.

[50] Nordfors K, Haapasalo J, Korja M, Niemelä A, Laine J, Parkkila AK, Pastorekova S, Pastorek J, Waheed A, Sly WS, Parkkila S, Haapasalo H (2010); The tumour-associated carbonic anhydrases CA II, CA IX and CA XII in a group of medulloblastomas and supratentorial primitive neuroectodermal tumours: an association of CA IX with poor prognosis. BMC Cancer. 18;10:148.

[51] Oosterwijk E, Ruiter DJ, Hoedemaeker PJ, Pauwels EK, Jonas U, Zwartendijk J, Warnaar SO (1986); Monoclonal antibody G 250 recognizes a determinant present in renal-cell carcinoma and absent from normal kidney. Int J Cancer 38:489-94.

[52] Opavský R, Pastoreková S, Zelník V, Gibadulinová A, Stanbridge EJ, Závada J, Kettmann R, Pastorek J (1996); Human MN/CA9 gene, a novel member of the carbonic anhydrase family: structure and exon to protein domain relationships. Genomics. 33:480-7.

[53] Parkkila AK, Herva R, Parkkila S, Rajaniemi H (1995); Immunohistochemical demonstration of human carbonic anhydrase isoenzyme II in brain tumours. Histochem J. 27:974-82.

[54] Parkkila S, Parkkila AK, Saarnio J, Kivelä J, Karttunen TJ, Kaunisto K, Waheed A, Sly WS, Türeci O, Virtanen I, Rajaniemi H (2000a); Expression of the membrane-associated carbonic anhydrase isozyme XII in the human kidney and renal tumors. J Histochem Cytochem. 48:1601-8.

[55] Parkkila S, Rajaniemi H, Parkkila AK, Kivela J, Waheed A, Pastoreková S, Pastorek J, Sly WS (2000b); Carbonic anhydrase inhibitor suppresses invasion of renal cancer cells in vitro. Proc. Natl. Acad. Sci. U S A 97:2220-4.

[56] Pastorek J, Pastoreková S, Callebaut I, Mornon JP, Zelník V, Opavsky R, Zat'ovicová M, Liao S, Portetelle D, Stanbridge EJ, Závada J, Burny A, Kettman R (1994); Cloning and characterization of MN, a human tumor-associated protein with a domain homologous to carbonic anhydrase and a putative helix- loop-helix DNA binding segment. Oncogene 9: 2877–2888.

[57] Pastoreková S, Parkkila S, Parkkila A-K, Opavský R, Zelnik V, Saarnio J, Pastorek J (1997); Carbonic anhydrase IX, MN/CA IX: Analysis of stomach complementary DNA sequence and expression in human and rat alimentary tracts. Gastroenterology 112:398-408.

[58] Pastoreková S, Parkkila S, Pastorek J, Supuran CT (2004); Carbonic anhydrases: current state of the art, therapeutic applications and future prospects. J. Enzyme Inhib. Med. Chem. 19:199-229.

[59] Pastoreková S, Parkkila S, Zavada J (2006); Tumor-associated carbonic anhydrases and their clinical significance. Adv. Clin. Chem. 42:167-216.

[60] Pastoreková S, Ratcliffe PJ, Pastorek J (2008); Molecular mechanisms of carbonic anhydrase IX-mediated pH regulation under hypoxia. BJU Int. 101:8-15.

[61] Pastoreková S, Závadová Z, Kost'ál M, Babusiková O, Závada J (1992); A novel quasi-viral agent, MaTu, is a two-component system. Virology 187:620-626.

[62] Pietilä S, Korpela R, Lenko HL, Haapasalo H, Alalantela R, Nieminen P, Koivisto AM, Mäkipernaa A (2012); Neurological outcome of childhood brain tumor survivors. J Neurooncol. 108:153-61.

[63] Pokhrel A and Hakulinen T (2009); Age-standardisation of relative survival ratios of cancer patients in a comparison between countries, genders and time periods. Eur J Cancer 45:642-647.

[64] Pollack IF, Jakacki RI (2011); Childhood brain tumors: epidemiology, current management and future directions. Nature Rev Neurol 7:495-506.

[65] Preusser M, Wolfsberger S, Haberler C, Breitschopf H, Czech T, Slavc I, Harris AL, Acker T, Budka H, Hainfellner JA. Vascularization and expression of hypoxia-related

tissue factors in intracranial ependymoma and their impact on patient survival (2005); Acta Neuropathol. 109:211-6.

[66] Proescholdt MA, Mayer C, Kubitza M, Schubert T, Liao SY, Stanbridge EJ, Ivanov S, Oldfield EH, Brawanski A, Merrill MJ (2005); Expression of hypoxia-inducible carbonic anhydrases in brain tumors. Neuro Oncol. 7:465-75.

[67] Proescholdt M, Merrill M, Stoerr EM, Lohmeier A, Dietmaier W, Brawanski A. Expression of carbonic anhydrase IX in craniopharyngiomas (2011); J Neurosurg. 115:796-801.

[68] Ramsey ML, Yuh BJ, Johnson MT, Yeldandi AV, Zynger DL. Carbonic anhydrase IX is expressed in mesothelioma and metastatic clear cell renal cell carcinoma of the lung (2012); Virchows Arch;460:89-93.

[69] Reimers TS, Ehrenfels S, Mortensen EL, Schmiegelow M, Sønderkaer S, Carstensen H, Schmiegelow K and Müller J (2003); Cognitive deficits in long-term survivors of childhood brain tumors: Identification of predictive factors. Med Pediatr Oncol 40:26-34.

[70] Robertson N, Potter C, Harris AL (2004); Role of carbonic anhydrase IX in human tumor cell growth, survival, and invasion. Cancer Res. 64:6160-5.

[71] Saarnio J, Parkkila S, Parkkila A-K, Haukipuro K, Pastoreková S, Pastorek J, Kairaluoma MI, Karttunen TJ (1998a); Immunohistochemical study of colorectal tumors for expression of a novel transmembrane carbonic anhydrase, MN/CA IX, with potential value as a marker of cell proliferation. Am. J. Pathol. 153: 279-285.

[72] Saarnio J, Parkkila S, Parkkila A-K, Waheed A, Casey MC, Zhou ZY, Pastoreková S, Pastorek J, Karttunen T, Haukipuro K, Kairaluoma MI, Sly WS (1998b); Immunohistochemistry of carbonic anhydrase isozyme IX (MN/CA IX) in human gut reveals polarized expression in the epithelial cells with the highest proliferative capacity. J. Histochem. Cytochem. 46: 497-504.

[73] Saarnio J, Parkkila S, Parkkila A-K, Pastoreková S, Haukipuro K, Pastorek J, Juvonen T, Karttunen TJ (2001); Transmembrane carbonic anhydrase, MN/CA IX, is a potential biomarker for biliary tumours. J. Hepatol. 35:643-649.

[74] Said HM, Hagemann C, Staab A, Stojic J, Kühnel S, Vince GH, Flentje M, Roosen K, Vordermark D (2007a); Expression patterns of the hypoxia-related genes osteopontin, CA9, erythropoietin, VEGF and HIF-1alpha in human glioma in vitro and in vivo. Radiother Oncol. 83:398-405.

[75] Said HM, Staab A, Hagemann C, Vince GH, Katzer A, Flentje M, Vordermark D (2007b); Distinct patterns of hypoxic expression of carbonic anhydrase IX (CA IX) in human malignant glioma cell lines. J. Neurooncol 81:27-38.

[76] Said HM, Polat B, Staab A, Hagemann C, Stein S, Flentje M, Theobald M, Katzer A, Vordermark D (2008); Rapid detection of the hypoxia-regulated CA-IX and NDRG1 gene expression in different glioblastoma cells in vitro. Oncol Rep. 20:413-9.

[77] Sandlund J, Oosterwijk E, Grankvist K, Oosterwijk-Wakka J, Ljungberg B, Rasmuson T (2007); Prognostic impact of carbonic anhydrase IX expression in human renal cell carcinoma. BJU Int. 100:556-60.

[78] Sathornsumetee S, Cao Y, Marcello JE, Herndon JE 2nd, McLendon RE, Desjardins A, Friedman HS, Dewhirst MW, Vredenburgh JJ, Rich JN (2008); Tumor angiogenic and hypoxic profiles predict radiographic response and survival in malignant astrocytoma patients treated with bevacizumab and irinotecan. J. Clin. Oncol. 26:271-8.

[79] Sly WS, Hu PY (1995); Human carbonic anhydrases and carbonic anhydrase deficiencies. Annu. Rev. Biochem. 64:375-401.

[80] Statistics Finland (2011); Statistical databases for cause of death in years 2003-2009.

[81] Stupp R, Hegi ME, Mason WP, van den Bent MJ, Taphoorn MJ, Janzer RC, Ludwin SK, Allgeier A, Fisher B, Belanger K, Hau P, Brandes AA, Gijtenbeek J, Marosi C, Vecht CJ, Mokhtari K, Wesseling P, Villa S, Eisenhauer E, Gorlia T, Weller M, Lacombe D, Cairncross JG, Mirimanoff RO; European Organisation for Research and Treatment of Cancer Brain Tumour and Radiation Oncology Groups; National Cancer Institute of Canada Clinical Trials Group (2009); Effects of radiotherapy with concomitant and adjuvant temozolomide versus radiotherapy alone on survival in glioblastoma in a randomised phase III study: 5-year analysis of the EORTC-NCIC trial. Lancet Oncol. 10:459-66.

[82] Svastová E, Zilka N, Zat'ovicová M, Gibadulinová A, Ciampor F, Pastorek J, Pastoreková S (2003); Carbonic anhydrase IX reduces E-cadherin-mediated adhesion of MDCK cells via interaction with beta-catenin. Exp. Cell. Res. 290:332-45.

[83] Swietach P, Wigfield S, Supuran CT, Harris AL, Vaughan-Jones RD (2008); Cancer-associated, hypoxia-inducible carbonic anhydrase IX facilitates CO2 diffusion. BJU Int. 101:22-4.

[84] Swinson DE, Jones JL, Richardson D, Wykoff C, Turley H, Pastorek J, Taub N, Harris AL, O'Byrne KJ (2003); Carbonic anhydrase IX expression, a novel surrogate marker of tumor hypoxia, is associated with a poor prognosis in non-small-cell lung cancer. J Clin Oncol. 21:473-82.

[85] Turner JR, Odze RD, Crum CP, Resnick MB (1997); MN antigen expression in normal, preneoplastic, and neoplastic esophagus: a clinicopathological study of a new cancer-associated biomarker. Hum. Pathol. 28: 740-744.

[86] Vermylen P, Roufosse C, Burny A, Verhest A, Bosschaerts T, Pastoreková S, Ninane V, Sculier JP (1999); Carbonic anhydrase IX antigen differentiates between preneoplastic malignant lesions in non-small lung carcinoma. Eur Respir J. 14:806-11.

[87] Wykoff CC, Beasley NJ, Watson PH, Turner KJ, Pastorek J, Sibtain A, Wilson GD, Turley H, Talks KL, Maxwell PH, Pugh CW, Ratcliffe PJ, Harris AL (2000); Hypoxia-inducible expression of tumor-associated carbonic anhydrases. Cancer Res. 60:7075-83.

[88] Yoo H, Baia GS, Smith JS, McDermott MW, Bollen AW, Vandenberg SR, Lamborn KR, Lal A.Expression of the hypoxia marker carbonic anhydrase 9 is associated with anaplastic phenotypes in meningiomas (2007); Clin Cancer Res. 13:68-75.

[89] Yoo H, Sohn S, Nam BH, Min HS, Jung E, Shin SH, Gwak HS, Lee SH (2010); The expressions of carbonic anhydrase 9 and vascular endothelial growth factor in astrocytic tumors predict a poor prognosis. Int J Mol Med. 26:3-9.

[90] Závada J, Závadová Z, Pastoreková S, Ciampor F, Pastorek J, Zelník V (1993); Expression of MaTu-MN protein in human tumor cultures and in clinical specimens. Int J Cancer. 54:268-74.

Radioresistance of Brain Tumors

In silico Analysis of Transcription Factors Associated to Differentially Expressed Genes in Irradiated Glioblastoma Cell Lines

P. R. D. V. Godoy, S. S. Mello, F. S. Donaires,
E. A. Donadi, G. A. S. Passos and
E. T. Sakamoto-Hojo

Additional information is available at the end of the chapter

1. Introduction

Glioblastoma multiforme (GBM) is one of the most frequent tumors in the central nervous system and the most malignant tumor among gliomas. In the past two decades, cytogenetic and molecular genetic studies have identified a number of recurrent chromosomal abnormalities and genetic alterations in malignant gliomas, particularly in GBM [1]. It was already described that GBM harbors combinations of the following genetic alterations: loss of heterozygozity of 10q, *EGFR* amplification, *TP53* mutations, p16^{INK4a} deletion and PTEN mutations [2]. New integrative genomics studies provided a comprehensive view of the complicated genomic landscape of GBM, revealing a set of core signaling pathways commonly activated in GBM involving TP53, RB, and RTK (receptor tyrosine kinase) pathways [3, 4]. The majority of GBM tumors present genetic alterations in all three pathways, which helps to stimulate cell proliferation and enhance cell survival while allowing tumor cells to escaping from cell-cycle checkpoints, senescence, and apoptosis. This approach also identified previously unknown genetic alterations in *IDH1/2*, *NF1*, *ERBB2*, and *NFKBIA* genes [1].

The current GBM treatment involves aggressive management including surgery, adjuvant temozolomide-based chemotherapy, and radiotherapy [5], but GBM patients still present a dismal prognosis, and the median survival is 14.6 months from diagnosis [6]. Although radiotherapy has been found to significantly prolong survival rates for GBM patients, radioresistance is a typical characteristic of this tumor [7].

Current genome-wide studies and the molecular characterization of GBM have allowed the identification of potential new targets, development of novel therapeutic small molecules and monoclonal antibodies and initiation of clinical trials with these targets [6, 8-10]. However, there is a wide molecular diversity and heterogeneity associated with the aberrantly GBM signaling pathways, culminating in the relative lack of success of these new approaches [10]. Recently, an alternative strategy involves the selective targeting of GBM stem cells, which are resistant to chemo- and radiotherapy. But still, almost all small-molecule inhibitors designed to target these cells failed to demonstrate the effectiveness of this strategy, compared with the conventional therapy [11].

Considering that most of the treatment protocols are still ineffective, novel approaches are needed towards killing of GBM cells. Transcription machinery, as well as its regulatory elements is also a feasible new target for the application of molecular therapies. Transcription of DNA is dependent on the spatially and temporally coordinated interaction between transcriptional machinery involving RNA polymerase II, transcription factors (TFs)) and transcriptional regulatory components (promoter elements, enhancers, silencers and locus control regions) [12, 13]. The low level of transcription, directed by the general transcription factors associated to RNA polymerase core enzyme, is known as basal transcription [14]. However, there is a rapidly expanding number of 'context-dependent' transcription factors that bind DNA and these TFs are capable of positively or negatively regulating the transcription process depending on the context of their binding sites, the complement of protein interactions and other environmental influences [15].

Postgenomic analyses of major transcription factor families, in both malignant and nonmalignant cell types, have opened new discussions about TF function. The mechanisms by which TFs act in cancer cell systems appear to exhibit a restricted repertoire of skills and plasticity displayed by normal cell systems [16]. The evolution of a restricted malignant transcriptome can be seen clearly in the nuclear receptor superfamily, but is also apparent in the MYC and AP-1 networks [17]. Oncogenic transcriptional rigidity reflects the simultaneous deregulation of target loci such that proliferative and survival signals are enhanced and antimitotic inputs are either limited or lost. Co-repressor proteins significantly contribute with the disruption of these processes [16]. Therefore, understanding mechanisms involved in gene regulation and transcriptional network may lead to a better knowledge about the crucial functions of TFs, providing information to explore possibilities of their application as molecular targets in cancer therapy [18].

A valuable tool to study the transcription machinery is the DNA microarray technology [19], which measures the transcript expression of thousands of genes to identify changes in expression profiles at different biological conditions [20-24], thus allowing to compare different cell types under diverse treatment conditions. The influence of *TP53* status on transcriptional profiles was previously described in tumor cell lines [25, 26]. Expression signatures of irradiated GBM cells were already performed for cell lines that are proficient and deficient for *TP53* [27, 28].

Recently, information on the regulation of gene expression can also be used within the context of functional enrichment tests, and different databases containing TFs binding sites and other regulatory motifs are available, allowing to scan promoter regions of genes to detect the presence of target motifs [29]. This information allow to determining whether a set of pre-selected genes is under control of TFs. FatiGO + [30] is a web-based tool capable of associating TFs that are common to a gene set used as parameters. This TF prediction method was already applied to a GBM dataset obtained from public repositories of microarray experiments, and the up-regulation of two predicted TFs, E2F1 and E2F4, was validated for several GBM cell lines [31], demonstrating the suitability of this method.

In the current study, we aimed to identify TFs that could be predicted from significant differentially expressed genes (previously obtained in microarray experiments in irradiated GBM cells) using an *in silico* analysis.

We found few predicted TFs that were common between GBM cell lines, while several exclusive TFs were found for each cell line, indicating that the transcriptional response to ionizing radiation is very particular to each cell line examined in our microarray study, a fact that can be due to the genetic heterogeneity inherent to GBM cells. In spite of this, there was a convergence of biological functions among cell lines; the most relevant processes were related to apoptosis, cell proliferation, cell cycle, DNA repair, oxidative stress, among others. Furthermore, the present results also showed several TFs that were already reported as associated to cancer and stress responses.

2. Materials and methods

2.1. Briefly characterization of the experiment that provided the statistically modulated genes used for TF prediction

2.1.1. Cell culture and irradiation

Human GBM T98G and U87MG cell lines were supplied by the American Type Culture Collection (ATCC) (Rockville, Maryland, USA) and gently donated by Dr. Mari C. Sogayar (Universidade de São Paulo, Brazil). U343MG-a (U343), a cell line established from a primary malignant astrocytoma in an adult [32], was kindly donated by Dr. James T. Rutka (The Arthur and Sonia Labatt Brain Tumour Research Center, Canada); U251MG cell lines was also purchased from the ATCC (Rockville, MD, USA) and gently donated by Dr. Guido Lenz (Universidade Federal do Rio Grande do Sul, Brazil) [33]. All cell lines grown in the presence of DMEM + HAM F10 medium (Sigma-Aldrich, St. Louis, USA) plus 10% fetal calf serum (Cultilab, Campinas, Brazil), and kept at 37°C and 5% CO2, until they reach semi-confluency. Cells were sub-cultured and 1×10^6 cells were seeded in 25 cm^2 flasks, being incubated at 37°C for 48 h, and irradiated with 8 Gy of gamma-rays (^{60}Co source, dose rate of 2.0 Gy / min., Unit Gammatron S-80, Siemens, 1.25 MeV, HC-FMRP/USP).

2.1.2. cDNA microarrays method and analysis

Two experiments with irradiated and sham-irradiated GBM cells were carried out using a glass slide microarrays containing ~4300 clones of cDNA probe (in replicates) from the human IMAGE Consortium cDNA library [34]; kindly provided by Dr. Catherine Nguyen (IN-SERM-CNRS, Marseille, France)], and prepared according to the protocol described by Hegde et al [35]. Microarrays were spotted onto glass slides (Corning, Lowell, MA, USA) by using a Generation III Array Spotter (Amersham Molecular Dynamics, Sunnyvale, USA) according to the manufacturer's instructions.

Total RNA extraction was performed for all cell lines, 30 min. and 6 h after irradiation, using the Trizol reagent (Invitrogen, Carlsbad, USA) according to manufacturer's instructions. Each cDNA sample was spotted twice in the slide (duplicate spots). The cDNA complex probes were prepared using the CyScribe Post Labeling Kit (Amersham Biosciences, Buckinghamshire, UK) as previously described [23]. Hybridizations were carried out using an automatic system (Automatic Slide Processor, Amersham Biosciences, UK) and signals were immediately captured after the final wash procedure, using a Generation III laser scanner (Amersham Biosciences, UK). This array platform was already used in several studies [22-26, 36].

2.1.3. Data acquisition and gene expression analysis

The provided microarray data was filtered and normalized [25, 36]. Following the normalization procedure, microarray data was exported to tab-delimited tables in MEV format and analyzed in MEV (v. 3.1) software [37].

The gene set submitted to SAM (Significance Analysis of Microarray [20]) were previously obtained by a t-test (α=5%) comparing irradiated (8 Gy) *versus* unirradiated (controls) T98G, U251MG, U343MG-a and U87MG cell lines, separately, considering two time points (30 min. and 6 h). The overall results are displayed in Table 1. The complete gene lists are available at http//www.rge.fmrp.usp.br/passos/genesgbm01/

Condition	Number of genes		Fold Change variation
	up-regulated	down-regulated	
U343MG-a (30 min.)	7	116	+1.53 to -2.42
U343MG-a (6 h)	3	11	+1.83 to -1.39
U87MG (30 min.)	56	73	+1.88 to - 2.95
U87MG (6 h)	86	54	+1.68 to -1.95
T98G (30 min)	32	0	+2.26 to +1.13
T98G (6 h)	16	7	+2.70 to -1.63
U251MG (30 min.)	12	69	+1.85 to -1.40
U251MG (6 h)	17	20	+2.28 to -2.18

Table 1. Overall quantitative results on significant differentially expressed genes obtained by the DNA microarray method, and analysis performed by SAM – Significance Analysis of Microarray (FDR < 5 %), for the comparison irradiated *versus* un-irradiated cells.RNA samples from U87, U343, T98 and U251 cells were collected at 30 min. and 6 h following irradiation with 8 Gy of gamma-rays. Fold-change (+) or (-) means up- and down-regulation in transcript expression, respectively.

The list of significantly modulated genes was obtained for a FDR < 5%. U343 cells showed 123 and 14 significantly differentially expressed genes at 30 min and 6 h after irradiation, respectively, whereas U87 showed 129 genes at 30 min and 140 genes at 6 h; T98G cell line displayed 32 and 23 significantly up-regulated genes at 30 min. and 6 h, respectively, whereas U251 showed 81 genes at 30 min. and 37 genes at 6 h (Table 2).

2.2. Transcriptional factor analysis

The analysis of TFs related to the significant differentially expressed genes (SAM) was performed by applying the FatiGO + [30]. This program uses the TRANSFAC [38], and CisRed [39] transcription factors database, including their respective binding sites and regulated genes.

FatiGO + analyzes if the pre –selected set of genes (provided after SAM analysis), are under control of the same TF, and search for significant enrichments to each TF that is associated to the gene list compared to the complete reference list, containing ~4300 clones that were spotted onto the microarray slide [29].

The p-values obtained in the analysis of regulatory elements have been established by the program using the Fisher's exact test for multiple comparisons (unadjusted p-value). The Enrichment Index (EI) calculated for each TF corresponds to the increment obtained regarding the number of genes (%) statistically modulated (SAM) that are associated to a specific TF (List #1) divided by the total number of genes (%) in the array set that were predicted as targets for the same TF (List #2):

EI = % gene List #1/ % gene list #2

The TFs were selected according to unadjusted p-values < 0.05. The genes were submitted to FatiGO + v3.2, using the Gene symbol identifier and the selected gene distance of 10 kb. After selecting the TFs associated to modulated genes (SAM), a search was conducted in PubMed (http://www.ncbi.nlm. Nih.gov / sites / entrez /) looking for biological functions of those TFs.

2.3. Quantitative real-time PCR (qPCR)

We analyzed the transcript expression of HEB, a predict TF that was found associated to 57.7% of up-regulated genes in U87 cells, 30 min. after IR. The reverse transcription step was carried out in the remaining RNA samples from microarray experiments, with the Superscript III Reverse Transcriptase kit (Invitrogen, USA), according to manufacturer's instructions. The integrity of cDNA samples was validated by the amplification of the endogenous B2M gene and visualization in agarose gel electrophoresis. qPCR was carried out using SYBR green master mix (Applied Biosystems, Foster City, USA) and the expression levels were estimated by the Relative Expression Software Tool (REST) [49], using 10000 interactions as setup parameter. All primers (Integrated DNA Technologies, Coralville, USA) were designed in Primer3 software [50] and are displayed on Table 2. The reactions were carried out in the Applied Biosystems 7500 Real-Time PCR System (Applied

Biosystems, USA) equipment, using primer sets with an annealing temperature near 60°C and an amplicon of 100–120 bp. The PCR cycle was the following: pre-heating at 50°C for 2 min., 10 min. at 95°C (denaturation step), followed by 40 cycles at 95°C for 15 sec., and at 60°C for 60 sec. The dissociation curves were set up as following: 95°C for 15 sec., 60°C for 20 sec. and 95°C for 15 sec.

Primer	Sequence	PCR product size (pb)
B2M – forward	5'- AGGCTATCCAGCGTACTCCA - 3'	112
B2M – reverse	5' - TCAATGTCGGATGGATGAAA - 3'	
HEB – forward	5' - CCGCTTGAGTTATCCTCCAC - 3'	116
HEB – reverse	5' - GTGAGGCAGCAACGTAAGGT - 3'	

Table 2. Primer sequences used in Real Time qPCR; the housekeeping B2M gene was used as internal control.

2.4. Western Blot (WB)

Protein extraction was performed with the Trizol reagent (Invitrogen, Carlsbad-USA) according to the manufacturer's instructions, using the same samples for RNA extraction. These samples were obtained from U87 cells collected at 30 min. post-irradiation. The expression of HEB was analyzed by Western blot, using ACTB as internal control. Samples were prepared with 30 µg of total protein. After electrophoresis, proteins were transferred from the gel to the membrane Invitrolon PVDF using the XCell IITM Blot Module system (Invitrogen, Carlsbad - USA). The immunodetection and protein visualization were conducted with the WesternBreeze Chromogenic kit (Invitrogen, Carlsbad - USA). The antibodies used in this study were anti-HEB (Santa Cruz, Santa Cruz, USA), and anti-ACTB (Cell Signaling, Danvers, USA), dilution of 1:1000.

We performed densitometric analysis of WB bands using the GelPro Analyzer (MediaCybernetics, Rockville, USA) 4.0, and the relative expression of HEB was calculated relatively to ACTB.

3. Results

In the FatiGO + analysis, the lists of statistically modulated genes (SAM) were up-loaded in order to find TFs that were significantly associated with up-regulated and down-regulated genes for non-adjusted p-values < 0.05 (Table 3).

A Venn diagram was constructed based on the numbers of predicted TFs from data set previously obtained for each cell line (microarray experiments) (Fig. 1). TFs predicted for 30 min and 6 h were pooled together. Each cell line showed a number of exclusive TFs, but we also observed common TFs between cell lines. Out of 18 exclusive TFs found for U87MG cell line, PEBP (p = 0.008), Bach2 (p = 0.007), Freac-4 (p = 0.003), HLV (p = 0.006), Evi-1 (p = 0.009) displayed the lowest p-values, while PPARG and SEF-1 displayed the highest EI (31.3). U343 presented 9 exclusive TFs; High values of EI were found for MAF (33.1), E2F:DP-1 (22.0), PR (45.5) and STAT3 (38.5), and ARP-1 was the TF presenting the lowest p-value (0.009). T98G cells displayed only 6 exclusive TFs: EBF, Pax, Pbx1b, C/EBP, Poly A downstream element and Pax-9; two of them, EBF and PolyA showed low p-values, 0.005 and 0.007, respectively. Regarding U251MG cells, 13 TFs were predicted, and only APOLYA presented a high EI (27.8) (Table 3).

Interestingly, STAT3 was the common TF found for TP53 wild-type cells; however, this TF was associated with up-regulated genes in U87, and with down-regulated genes in U343. Only one TF (VBP) was common among three cell lines (U87, U343 and U251), being associated with down-regulated genes. Among the *TP53* mutant cell lines, ATF4 was common between T98 and U251, associated with up-regulated genes (30 min. and 6 h). Two TFs were found common between U343 and U251, TEF (associated to down-regulated genes, 30 min.) and MAF (associated to up-regulated, 6 h). Finally, C/BPGamma was commonly predicted for up-regulated genes in U87 (30 min.) and U251 (6 h) cell lines (Fig. 1).

Therefore, our results showed that most of the predicted TFs were exclusive to each cell line and few TFs were common among the GBM cell lines; these results indicate that the transcriptional response to ionizing radiation is very particular to each cell line, and most probably this can be due to the genetic heterogeneity of GBM cells.

By using the real time qPCR method, we confirmed the expression of HEB to validate the *in silico* prediction for this TF. By using the REST 2009 software, we found that HEB was statistically up-regulated (+2.6) when comparing irradiated and sham-irradiated U87 cell lines (30 min.) (Fig. 2A). Primer efficiency was also determined for B2M (0.9615) and HEB (0.9652).

We also look for HEB protein expression by Western Blot; both ACTB and HEB antibodies were used for irradiated and sham-irrradiated U87, 30 min after irradiation (Fig.2B). The relative expression values calculated by densitometric analysis showed that HEB expression was 1.7 higher in irradiated (8 Gy) cells, relatively to the control value (Fig. 2C).

U343MG-a					
Collection time	Transcription factor	% of genes (List 1)	% of genes (List 2)	EI	p-value
30 min. (↓)	ARP-1	14.8	6.7	2.2	0.009
	TEF	37.5	25.3	1.5	0.013
	VBP	19.3	10.4	1.9	0.013
	Imperfect Hogness/Goldberg BOX	2.3	0.2	14.2	0.016
	Muscle initiator sequence-20	20.5	12.2	1.7	0.031

U343MG-a				
Collection time	Transcription factor	% of genes (List 1)	% of genes (List 2)	EI	p-value
	Elk-1	44.3	33.1	1.3	0.038
	Sox-5	4.6	1.5	3.1	0.048
	ACAAT	12.5	6.7	1.9	0.049
6 h (↑)	MAF	50.0	1.5	33.1	0.031
	E2F-4:DP-1	50.0	2.3	22.0	0.046
	ICSBP	40.0	3.7	10.9	0.013
6 h (↓)	PR	20.0	0.4	45.5	0.024
	STAT3	20.0	0.5	38.5	0.028
	ARP-1	40.0	6.7	6.0	0.040

U87 MG				
Collection time	Transcription factor	% of genes (List 1)	% of genes (List 2)	EI	p-value
	C/EBPgamma	85.0	64.4	1.3	0.007
	AP-1	80.0	61.1	1.3	0.014
	HEB	57.5	38.5	1.5	0.021
30 min. (↑)	SREBP-1	97.5	84.5	1.2	0.024
	FOXP3	87.5	72.0	1.2	0.032
	PPARG	2.5	0.1	31.3	0.046
	SEF-1	2.5	0.1	31.3	0.046
	Bach2	63.5	43.9	1.4	0.007
	PEBP	28.9	14.4	2.0	0.008
30 min. (↓)	COUP-TF:HNF-4	11.5	3.7	3.1	0.014
	MEF-3	5.8	1.2	5.0	0.026
	FOX	78.9	64.8	1.2	0.039
6 h (↑)	DEC	45.6	31.9	1.4	0.032
	STAT3	3.5	0.5	6.8	0.042
	Freac-4	10.5	1.6	6.8	0.003
	HLF	50.0	28.2	1.8	0.006
6 h (↓)	Evi-1	97.4	81.6	1.2	0.009
	VBP	23.7	10.4	2.3	0.015
	TCF-4	55.3	37.2	1.5	0.028

U343MG-a					
Collection time	**Transcription factor**	**% of genes (List 1)**	**% of genes (List 2)**	**EI**	**p-value**
	AP-1	79.0	61.1	1.3	0.028
	Gfi-1	10.5	3.1	3.4	0.031
	CRE-BP1	15.8	6.6	2.4	0.039
	HNF-4alpha	29.0	16.4	1.8	0.047

T98G					
Collection time	**Transcription factor**	**% of genes (List 1)**	**% of genes (List 2)**	**EI**	**p-value**
30 min. (↑)	EBF	29.6	10.5	2.8	0.005
	ATF4	22.2	8.4	2.6	0.023
	Pax	92.6	75.3	1.2	0.041
6 h (↑)	Pbx1b	14.3	1.8	8.2	0.026
6 h (↓)	C/EBP	100.0	20.0	5.0	0.002
	Poly A downstream element	75.0	12.6	6.0	0.007
	Pax-9	75.0	23.8	3.2	0.045

U251MG					
Collection time	**Transcription factor**	**% of genes (List 1)**	**% of genes (List 2)**	**EI**	**p-value**
30 min. (↑)	SMAD-4	40.0	10.4	3.9	0.015
	PTF1-beta	20.0	2.7	7.4	0.030
	APOLYA	10.0	0.4	27.8	0.039
30 min. (↓)	VBP	21.7	10.4	2.1	0.025
	HNF-6	6.5	1.4	4.7	0.030
	E2F	52.2	36.0	1.4	0.030
	TEF	39.1	25.3	1.5	0.040
	TTF1	23.9	13.3	1.8	0.047
	CDP CR1	54.4	39.7	1.4	0.049
	POU1F1	54.4	39.7	1.4	0.049
6 h (↑)	MAF	15.4	1.5	10.2	0.017
	CREB	46.2	17.8	2.6	0.018
	ATF4	30.8	8.4	3.7	0.020
	MEIS1B:HOXA9	15.4	1.9	8.2	0.025

	U343MG-a				
Collection time	Transcription factor	% of genes (List 1)	% of genes (List 2)	EI	p-value
	C/EBPgamma	92.3	64.4	1.4	0.041
6 h (↓)	HES1	45.5	15.6	2.9	0.019
	Lmo2 complex	27.3	6.0	4.5	0.026
	ATATA	18.2	2.9	6.2	0.041

Table 3. Transcription factors associated with statistically modulated genes (SAM, FDR ≤ 5 %), as predicted by the FATIGO + v3.2., analysis performed for U343MG-a, U87MG, T98G and U251MG cell lines (30 min. and 6 h post-irradiation). We used gene lists that showed patterns of repression (↓) and induction (↑) in irradiated cells compared with mock-irradiated. The Enrichment Index (EI) calculated for each TF corresponds to the increment regarding the number of genes (%) statistically modulated (SAM) that are associated to a specific TF (List #1) divided by the total number of genes (%) in the array set that were predicted as targets for the same TF (List #2). The gene distance for the analysis of the TFs was 10 kb.

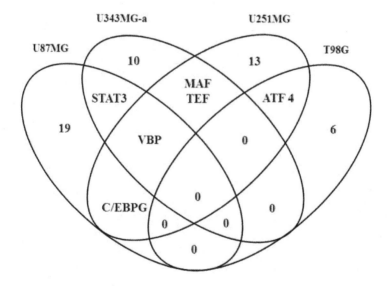

Figure 1. Venn diagram showing predicted TFs associated with significant differentially expressed genes (from micro-array experiments) selected for four GBM cell lines, comparing irradiated *versus* sham-irradiated cells, collected at 30 min. and 6 h following irradiation. TF prediction was carried out using FatiGO + v3.2.

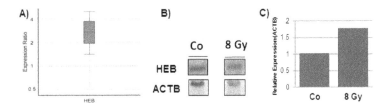

Figure 2. HEB expression. A) HEB expression levels obtained by the qPCR method. This TF was found associated with up-regulated genes in U87 cells, 30 min. after irradiation. Boxes represent the interquartile range; the dotted line represents the median value; whiskers represent the minimum and maximum observations. B) Protein expression analyzed by Western Blot using antibodies for HEB (Santa Cruz) and ACTB (Cell Signalling) as endogenous control. C) Densitometric analysis of Western Blot bands using the Gel Pro Analyzer 4.0 software displayed for HEB expression relatively to ACTB.

4. Discussion

Recently, genome wide technologies, such as DNA microarrays, provide a huge amount of information about gene expression, but require additional bioinformatics analyses for data interpretation. In order to reduce complex signatures to a small number of activated transcriptional elements, new bioinformatics tools have been developed. To date, genome-wide TF-binding regions and sites were identified using a variety of indirect methods and data sets, revealing abundant binding sites for different TFs in mammalian cells [40-43]. Using lists of differentially expressed genes that were generated by microarray experiments, it is possible to predict TFs that can target common binding sites to a gene set. In the current study, we performed an *in silico* analysis (FatiGO + v3.2.) to identify TFs from a list of significant differentially expressed genes selected for irradiated GBM cell lines in microarray experiments. Only few predicted TFs were common to GBM cell lines, while several TFs were exclusive to each cell line, indicating that the transcriptional response to ionizing radiation is very peculiar to each cell line examined in our microarray study. The most relevant predicted TFs are discussed below. While few predicted TFs were shared between different cell lines, several TFs were found exclusive to each cell line, except U251.

4.1. Commonly predicted TFs for two or three GBM cell lines

We found few TFs that were predicted for more than one cell line: MAF, TEF, ATF4, STAT3, VBP and C/EBPGamma. Most of these TFs (STAT3, TEF and VBP) are related to apoptosis, while other biological classes were also found, such as oxidative stress (ATF4), differentiation (MAF) and nucleotide excision repair (C/EBPGamma).

STAT3, *signal transducer and activator of transcription 3* (acute-phase response factor), is part of the STAT family of cytoplasmic latent transcription factors, and was predicted for the TP53 wild type cells, U87 (up-regulated genes, 6 h) and U343 (down-regulated genes, 6 h).

Phosphorylated STAT3 leads to transcriptional activation of downstream genes involved in processes such as cell proliferation, suppression of apoptosis, and angiogenesis [44, 45]. It was demonstrated that STAT3 is constitutively activated and overexpressed in human gliomas; STAT3 activation correlates with malignancy [46, 47], while STAT3 inhibition reduces the lethality of GBM tumors *in vivo* [48], and its inhibition have been tested in phase 0 trial in head and neck cancers [49].

Thyrotroph embryonic factor (TEF) and human hepatic leukemia factor (HLF) are members of the PAR (*proline and acidic amino acid-rich*) subfamily of basic region/leucine zipper (bZIP) transcription factors. The chicken vitellogenin gene-binding protein (VBP) is also a bZIP TF member and is considered as the chicken homologue of TEF. TEF was predicted from down-regulated genes in U343 and U251 (30 min.), and its homolog, VBP, from down-regulated genes in U87 (6 h), U343 (30 min.) and U251 (30 min.). PAR bZIP proteins have recently been shown to be involved in amino acid and neurotransmitter metabolism in both liver and brain [50]. PAR bZIP proteins are also able to transactivate the promoter of bcl-gS which is directly involved in apoptosis induction. Consistently, transfection of TEF induces the expression of endogenous bcl-gS in cancer cells, independently on TP53 [51].

Activating transcription factor 4 (*tax-responsive enhancer element B67*); activating transcription factor 4C (ATF4) belongs to the large ATF/CREB family of transcription factors [52] and was predicted from up-regulated genes in T98 (30 min) and U251 (6 h). Up-regulation of ATF4 is directly involved in the endoplasmic reticulum (ER) stress through induction of CHOP in GBM treated with Nelfinavir (protease inhibitor class of drugs) [53] or in concert with PERK, GADD34 and EIF2alpha in Hela cells submitted to hypoxia [54]. Therefore, activation of ATF4 was already reported in GBM treated cells.

MAF, the v-maf musculoaponeurotic fibrosarcoma oncogene homolog (avian) is a unique subclass of bZIP proteins and was predicted from up-regulated genes in U343 and U251 at 6 h. Depending on the binding site and binding partner, the encoded protein can be a transcriptional activator or repressor. Members of the MAF family appear to play important roles in the regulation of differentiation [55]. MAF was found up-regulated in various cancers, such as colon cancer (but only in tumors that presented high levels of COX-2 expression) [56], a small subset of myelomas, hairy cell leukemia, T- and NK-cell neoplasms and small cell lymphomas [57].

C/EBPGamma, a member of the CCAAT/enhancer-binding protein (C/EBP) family of transcription factors was predicted from up-regulated genes in U87 (30 min.) and U251 (6 h). This TF regulates the expression of ERCC5 [58], and is a participant of DNA repair [59], particularly in the nucleotide excision repair [60].

The predicted TFs represent the overall GBM response to irradiation, since they were selected for more than one cell line, and as mentioned above, their functions are directly associated with stress responses involving apoptosis, DNA repair and ER stress. Moreover, as an example of STAT3, which is in clinical trial [49], predicted TFs may constitute potential targets to be investigated and validated in cancer treatment.

4.2. Exclusively predicted TFs for irradiated U343 cell line

Few predicted TFs (PR, E2F4:DP-1, and ARP-1) associated with statistically significant modulated genes in irradiated U343 cells were found exclusive to this cell line. The functions of these TFs are mainly associated with cell cycle/ tumor growth, being involved in various types of cancer. The overexpression of E2F4 and its binding partner DP-1 revealed a dual function of E2F4, which acts as an activator as well as a repressor, being implicated in positive regulation of the cell cycle [61]. In a previous work, the up-regulation of E2F4 was confirmed for several GBM cell lines [31], demonstrating the potential of this TF as molecular target in cancer therapy.

Progesterone receptor (PR), a nuclear receptor transcription factor was associated with down-regulated genes in U343 cells (6 h). Steroid hormones participate in several physiological and pathological processes in the brain, including the regulation of tumor cell growth [62-64]. Progesterone exerts many of its effects by the interaction with specific intracellular receptors [62, 65].

ARP-1, also known as orphan nuclear receptor chicken ovalbumin upstream promoter transcription factor II (COUP-TFII) is a member of the steroid/thyroid nuclear hormone receptor superfamily [66] and can act as transcriptional repressor or activator. ARP-1 plays critical roles in organogenesis [67-70], and is a major angiogenesis regulator within the tumor microenvironment during pancreatic tumor progression and metastasis [71]. Besides, ARP-1 was associated with therapy response in oligodendroglial tumors with 1p/19q loss [72]. In the present study, this TF was predicted from down-regulated genes (30 min. and 6 h), indicating its possible involvement in radiation responses restricted to U343 cell line.

4.3. Exclusively predicted TFs for irradiated U87 cell line

A high number of TFs with low p-value (Bach2, PEBP, Freac-4, HLF and Evi-1) and high EI (PPARG and SEF-1) was associated with significant expressed genes in U87 cell line.

PPARG is a member of the peroxisome proliferator activated receptor (PPAR) family, a subfamily of the nuclear receptor superfamily [73]. The protein level of this receptor has been recently identified as a significant prognostic marker [74]. Interestingly, recent studies have shown that PPARG is expressed in normal and malignant human brain, and the treatment with PPARG agonists induces growth arrest and apoptosis in brain tumor cells *in vitro* and in animal models *in vivo* [75-77]. Recent findings show that PPARG agonists regulate growth and expansion of brain tumor stem cells [78] and also altered the expression of stemness genes [79]. Unfortunately, clinical trials also failed to demonstrate the effectiveness of such agonists as a monotherapy for cancer treatment, a fact which stimulates the search for combination treatments to enhance their effects [80].

Basic leucine zipper transcription factor 2 (Bach2) is an evolutionarily related member of the BTB-basic region leucine zipper transcription factor family. Bach2 can function as transcriptional activator and repressor [81]. This TF down-regulates cell proliferation of the neuroblastoma cell line N1E-115 and negatively affects their potential to differentiate, being considered as gatekeeper of the differentiated status [82]. Bach2 presents high frequency of loss of heterozygosity of the Bach2 gene in human B cell lymphomas [83]. Consistent with its putative role as a tumor suppressor, Bach2 enhances apoptosis in response to oxidative stress [84, 85].

The transcription Factor PEBP, also called Raf kinase inhibitor protein (RKIP) is a member of the phosphatidylethanolamine-binding protein (PEBP) family. RKIP plays a pivotal modulatory role in several protein kinase signaling cascades. RKIP regulates the activity of the Raf/MEK/ERK, which is responsible for proliferation and differentiation of diverse cell types [86]. It has been reported that RKIP was poorly expressed in primary tumors, being absent in various metastatic cancers; its induction sensitize resistant tumor cells to apoptosis by various chemo- and immunotherapeutic drugs, as well as inhibitors of metastasis [87].The absence of RKIP is also associated with highly malignant behavior and poor survival of patients [88].

The forkhead domain is a monomeric DNA binding motif that defines a rapidly growing family of eukaryotic transcriptional regulators. We found Freac-4, also known as Forkhead Box D1 (FOXD1) associated with down-regulated genes in U87 cells (6 h). This gene was found repressed in chemoresistant tumors, as analyzed by microarrays [89]. However, FOXD1 and FOXD2 were highly expressed in prostate cancer and lymph node metastases, among various cancer types [90]. In another study, using kidney-derived cell lines, it was suggested that FOXD1 may be regulated by TP53, WTAR (a mutated form of WT1) and WT1 [91].

As already mentioned, HLF is a member of PAR bZIP transcription factors, and was associated with down-regulated genes, 6 h after irradiation in U87. PAR bZIP proteins are also involved in apoptosis induction [51].The fused gene E2A-HLF was responsible for the development of lymphoid malignancies in 60 % of the transgenic mice [92].

Activator protein one (AP1) transcription factors are a family of jun and fos proteins, whose subunits present diverse pro/anti-cancer effects, like inhibition or increase in proliferation, inhibition of apoptosis and angiogenesis [93, 94]. AP-1 is one of the genes early activated after radiation in primary human B cells [95]. The inhibition of AP-1 blocks the proliferation of breast tumor cells by suppressing the growth factor signaling [96]. The modulation of AP-1 activity may be a new attempt to reduce the malignant transformation. However, only the function involved with malignancy should be targeted [97], since AP-1 presents oncogenic and anti-oncogenic properties. This TF was associated to U87 cells (up-regulated genes, 30 min.) and (down-regulated genes, 6 h).

The EVI1 gene encodes a zinc finger transcription factor with important roles in normal development and leukemogenesis. Reports in animal model and findings in *in vitro* studies. showed that EVI1 affected cellular proliferation, differentiation, and apoptosis [98]. EVI-1 was also found overexpressed in infratentorial ependymomas, it can promote proliferation of ependymal tumor cells, and its expression indicates an unfavorable prognosis [99].

U87 cell line presented several predicted TFs with significant p values and higher enrichment index than other cell lines. Most of the predicted TFs are related to apoptosis (PPARG, Batch2, PEBP, HLF, AP1 and EVI1), but they were associated with up- or down-regulated genes. Overall, the biological functions of these TFs are related to cell proliferation, differentiation and tumor growth, indicating the relevance of their deregulation in cancer development and malignancy, and possibly, in tumor responses to anti-cancer therapies.

4.4. Exclusively predicted TFs for irradiated T98G cell line

Only two TFs were predicted for T98G cells: EBF and C/EBP. The early B-cell factors (EBF) are a family of four highly conserved DNA-binding transcription factors with an atypical zinc-finger and helix-loop-helix motif. Zardo and colleagues found that the EBF3 locus on the human chromosome 10q is deleted or methylated in brain tumors [100]. Functional studies revealed that EBF3 activates genes involved in cell cycle arrest and apoptosis, while in opposite, it represses genes involved in cell survival and proliferation [101]. Therefore, EBFs represent a novel tumor suppressor whose inactivation blocks normal development and contributes to tumorigenesis of diverse types of human cancer [102].

CEBP is also known as basic leucine zipper transcription factor, CCAAT/enhancer binding protein alpha (CEBPA), which directly interacts with CDK2 and CDK4 and arrests cell proliferation by inhibition of these kinases [103]. CEBPA is crucial for normal granulopoiesis, and dominant-negative mutations of CEBPA gene were found in patients with myeloblastic subtypes (M1 and M2) of acute myeloid leukemia [104]. CEBPA also plays a role in DNA damage response dependent on TP53, as observed in keratinocytes [105]. C/EBPA was found silenced in human squamous cell carcinoma (SCC), and loss of C/EBPA confers susceptibility to UVB-induced skin SCCs involving defective cell cycle arrest in response to UVB [106]. Interestingly, these findings indicate the role of CEBP in DNA damage responses, and possibly, the potential of this TF to be explored as therapeutic molecular target.

4.5. Validation of TF prediction

As a predicted TF associated with up-regulated genes, HEB (p-value = 0.021 and EI = 1.5) was chosen to be studied in terms of expression levels, aiming to validate the *in silico* analysis, although for a single TF. Interestingly, we showed that HEB transcript expression was up-regulated (+2.6) in irradiated U87 cell line, 30 min. after irradiation, while HEB protein expression analyzed by Western blot was 1.7 higher in irradiated (8 Gy) cells, relatively to un-exposed controls.

HEB is a member of the class A basic helix-loop-helix (bHLH) family that participates in the nervous system development [107, 108]. According to O'Neil et al. [109], the repression of E47/HEB has been associated with the induction of leukemia in mice. In another study, it was demonstrated the induction of HEB in gliomas compared with non-neoplastic brain tissue [110]. Moreover, HEB seems to be involved in cell proliferation control of neural stem cells and also progenitor cells, being important to sustain their undifferentiated state during embryonic and adult neurogenesis [108]. Although HEB expression has not yet been correlated with radiation responses in GBM cells, in the present study, we found its association with significant differentially expressed genes at 30 min. following irradiation in U87 cell line; interestingly, we also showed that HEB transcript and protein expression was induced in irradiated U87 cell line, 30 min. after irradiation. This finding, although restrict to one TF, indicates the validity of the TF prediction by *in silico* analysis.

5. Conclusions: Lessons from TF prediction in irradiated GBM cells

The present findings about prediction of TFs associated to differentially expressed genes in GBM cell lines showed that few TFs were shared among different GBM cell lines, while several TFs were found exclusive to each cell line, indicating that the transcriptional response to ionizing radiation is very particular to each cell line, probably due to the genetic heterogeneity, which is characteristic of GBM cell lines. In spite of this observation, several biological functions were similar among cell lines, such as apoptosis, cell proliferation, cell cycle control, DNA repair, ER stress, and differentiation. Furthermore, most of the predicted TFs were already reported as differentially expressed, deleted or mutated in cancer, including GBM. However, apart the similarity of biological functions, different pathways seems to be associated to the predicted TFs. Interestingly, we could not find TP53 as a TF associated to the data set (List #1) analyzed in the present study, even for the GBM cells that were wild-type for *TP53* gene, and even considering the presence of *TP53* cDNA clone in the microarray slide. It is possible that the TP53 protein could not be activated in GBM cells, impairing its action as transcription factor, as previously suggested by other authors [111].

The most intriguing finding refers to apoptotic related TFs. Probably, predicted TFs related to apoptosis control, and found associated with expressed genes at early time (30 minutes) following irradiation, are related to survival in GBM cells; this is supported by reports showing that in general, these cells are very resistant to undergo apoptosis, even under conditions of drug treatment or radiation exposure [112-114]. In fact, GBM cells seem to be capable of activating several pathways to escaping from cell killing by anticancer therapies.

Even considering the relevance of our findings, some methodological limitations should be mentioned regarding *in silico* prediction of TFs. Despite the great advancement in terms of DNA binding sites detection, it is hard to determine which sites are functional regulatory elements that influence transcription. It is possible that a considerable fraction of these binding sites are nonfunctional and may constitute biological noise [115]. Other choices, such as ChIP experiments, may overcome this concern by detecting indirect TF-DNA interactions through protein/protein interaction [116].

In spite of the limitation mentioned above, in a previous study, we validated the expression of E2F [31] and the HEB expression was confirmed in the present study, both of them in GBM cell lines. In addition, we selected predicted TFs that were associated with stress response genes, and importantly, the TFs were reported as deregulated or mutated in different cancer types, thus indicating the relevance of further studies to better exploring the role of TFs in the context of therapeutic strategies based on molecular targets.

Author details

P. R. D. V. Godoy[1], S. S. Mello[1], F. S. Donaires[1], E. A. Donadi[2], G. A. S. Passos[3] and
E. T. Sakamoto-Hojo[1,4]

1 Department of Genetics, Faculty of Medicine, University of São Paulo, Ribeirão Preto, SP,
Brazil

2 Department of Medic Clinic, Faculty of Medicine, University of São Paulo, Ribeirão Preto,
SP, Brazil

3 Department of Genetics, Faculty of Medicine and Faculty of Dentistry, University of São
Paulo, Ribeirão Preto, SP, Brazil

4 Department of Biology, Faculty of Philosophy, Sciences and Letters-USP, University of São
Paulo, Ribeirão Preto, SP, Brazil

References

[1] Chen, J, RM McKay, and LF Parada, Malignant glioma: lessons from genomics, mouse models, and stem cells. Cell, 2012. 149(1): p. 36-47.

[2] Ohgaki, H, Genetic pathways to glioblastomas. Neuropathology, 2005. 25(1): p. 1-7.

[3] McLendon, R et al., Comprehensive genomic characterization defines human glioblastoma genes and core pathways. Nature, 2008. 455(7216): p. 1061-8.

[4] Parsons, DW, et al., An integrated genomic analysis of human glioblastoma multiforme. Science, 2008. 321(5897): p. 1807-12.

[5] Stupp, R, et al., Radiotherapy plus concomitant and adjuvant temozolomide for glioblastoma. N Engl J Med, 2005. 352(10): p. 987-96.

[6] Ohka, F, A Natsume, and T Wakabayashi, Current trends in targeted therapies for glioblastoma multiforme. Neurol Res Int, 2012. 2012: p. 878425.

[7] Stupp, R, et al., Chemoradiotherapy in malignant glioma: standard of care and future directions. J Clin Oncol, 2007. 25(26): p. 4127-36.

[8] Sathornsumetee, S, et al., Molecularly targeted therapy for malignant glioma. Cancer, 2007. 110(1): p. 13-24.

[9] Perry, J, et al., Novel therapies in glioblastoma. Neurol Res Int, 2012. 2012: p. 428565.

[10] Polivka, J, Jr., et al., New molecularly targeted therapies for glioblastoma multiforme. Anticancer Res, 2012. 32(7): p. 2935-46.

[11] Natsume, A, et al., Glioma-initiating cells and molecular pathology: implications for therapy. Brain Tumor Pathol, 2011. 28(1): p. 1-12.

[12] Thomas, MC and CM Chiang, The general transcription machinery and general co-factors. Crit Rev Biochem Mol Biol, 2006. 41(3): p. 105-78.

[13] Maston, GA, SK Evans, and MR Green, Transcriptional regulatory elements in the human genome. Annu Rev Genomics Hum Genet, 2006. 7: p. 29-59.

[14] Hampsey, M, Molecular genetics of the RNA polymerase II general transcriptional machinery. Microbiol Mol Biol Rev, 1998. 62(2): p. 465-503.

[15] Gaston, K and PS Jayaraman, Transcriptional repression in eukaryotes: repressors and repression mechanisms. Cell Mol Life Sci, 2003. 60(4): p. 721-41.

[16] Battaglia, S, O Maguire, and MJ Campbell, Transcription factor co-repressors in cancer biology: roles and targeting. Int J Cancer, 2010. 126(11): p. 2511-9.

[17] Thorne, JL, MJ Campbell, and BM Turner, Transcription factors, chromatin and cancer. Int J Biochem Cell Biol, 2009. 41(1): p. 164-75.

[18] Mees, C, J Nemunaitis, and N Senzer, Transcription factors: their potential as targets for an individualized therapeutic approach to cancer. Cancer Gene Ther, 2009. 16(2): p. 103-12.

[19] Kel, A, et al., Beyond microarrays: find key transcription factors controlling signal transduction pathways. BMC Bioinformatics, 2006. 7 Suppl 2: p. S13.

[20] Tusher, VG, R Tibshirani, and G Chu, Significance analysis of microarrays applied to the ionizing radiation response. Proc Natl Acad Sci U S A, 2001. 98(9): p. 5116-21.

[21] Sakamoto-Hojo, ET, et al., Gene expression profiles in human cells submitted to genotoxic stress. Mutat Res, 2003. 544(2 3): p. 403-13.

[22] Fachin, AL, et al., Gene expression profiles in human lymphocytes irradiated in vitro with low doses of gamma rays. Radiat Res, 2007. 168(6): p. 650-65.

[23] Fachin, AL, et al., Gene expression profiles in radiation workers occupationally exposed to ionizing radiation. J Radiat Res (Tokyo), 2009. 50(1): p. 61-71.

[24] Carminati, PO, et al., Alterations in gene expression profiles correlated with cisplatin cytotoxicity in the glioma U343 cell line. Genet Mol Biol, 2010. 33(1): p. 159-68.

[25] Godoy, PRDV, et al. Portrait of transcriptional expression profiles displayed by different glioblastoma cell lines. in: M Garami. (ed.) Molecular Targets of CNS Tumors. Rijeka: InTech; 2011. p. 277-300.

[26] da Silva, GN, et al., Expression of genes related to apoptosis, cell cycle and signaling pathways are independent of TP53 status in urinary bladder cancer cells. Mol Biol Rep, 2011. 38(6): p. 4159-70.

[27] Otomo, T, et al., Microarray analysis of temporal gene responses to ionizing radiation in two glioblastoma cell lines: up-regulation of DNA repair genes. J Radiat Res (Tokyo), 2004. 45(1): p. 53-60.

[28] Godoy, PRDV, et al., Glioblastoma cell lines differing in TP53 status (mutant or wild-type) display different molecular signaling responses to gamma-irradiation Submitted, 2013.

[29] Al-Shahrour, F, et al., FatiGO +: a functional profiling tool for genomic data. Integration of functional annotation, regulatory motifs and interaction data with microarray experiments. Nucleic Acids Res, 2007. 35(Web Server issue): p. W91-6.

[30] Al-Shahrour, F, et al., BABELOMICS: a suite of web tools for functional annotation and analysis of groups of genes in high-throughput experiments. Nucleic Acids Res, 2005. 33(Web Server issue): p. W460-4.

[31] Donaires, FS, et al., Transcriptional factors associated to over-expressed genes in glioblastoma multiforme, as predicted by in silico analysis on publicly microarray dataset Submitted, 2013.

[32] Dirks, PB, et al., Retinoic acid and the cyclin dependent kinase inhibitors synergistically alter proliferation and morphology of U343 astrocytoma cells. Oncogene, 1997. 15(17): p. 2037-48.

[33] Filippi-Chiela, EC, et al., Autophagy interplay with apoptosis and cell cycle regulation in the growth inhibiting effect of resveratrol in glioma cells. PLoS ONE, 2011. 6(6): p. e20849.

[34] Lennon, G, et al., The I.M.A.G.E. Consortium: An Integrated Molecular Analysis of Genomes and Their Expression. Genomics, 1996. 33(1): p. 151-152.

[35] Hegde, P, et al., A concise guide to cDNA microarray analysis. Biotechniques, 2000. 29(3): p. 548-50, 552-4, 556 passim.

[36] Mello, SS, et al., Delayed effects of exposure to a moderate radiation dose on transcription profiles in human primary fibroblasts. Environ Mol Mutagen, 2011. 52(2): p. 117-29.

[37] Saeed, AI, et al., TM4: a free, open-source system for microarray data management and analysis. Biotechniques, 2003. 34(2): p. 374-8.

[38] Wingender, E, et al., TRANSFAC: an integrated system for gene expression regulation. Nucleic Acids Res, 2000. 28(1): p. 316-9.

[39] Robertson, G, et al., cisRED: a database system for genome-scale computational discovery of regulatory elements. Nucleic Acids Res, 2006. 34(Database issue): p. D68-73.

[40] Ferretti, V, et al., PReMod: a database of genome-wide mammalian cis-regulatory module predictions. Nucleic Acids Res, 2007. 35(Database issue): p. D122-6.

[41] Bieda, M, et al., Unbiased location analysis of E2F1-binding sites suggests a wide-spread role for E2F1 in the human genome. Genome Res, 2006. 16(5): p. 595-605.

[42] Birney, E, et al., Identification and analysis of functional elements in 1% of the human genome by the ENCODE pilot project. Nature, 2007. 447(7146): p. 799-816.

[43] Cawley, S, et al., Unbiased mapping of transcription factor binding sites along human chromosomes 21 and 22 points to widespread regulation of noncoding RNAs. Cell, 2004. 116(4): p. 499-509.

[44] Bowman, T, et al., Stat3-mediated Myc expression is required for Src transformation and PDGF-induced mitogenesis. Proc Natl Acad Sci U S A, 2001. 98(13): p. 7319-24.

[45] Brennan, C, et al., Glioblastoma subclasses can be defined by activity among signal transduction pathways and associated genomic alterations. PLoS ONE, 2009. 4(11): p. e7752.

[46] Lo, HW, et al., Constitutively activated STAT3 frequently coexpresses with epidermal growth factor receptor in high-grade gliomas and targeting STAT3 sensitizes them to Iressa and alkylators. Clin Cancer Res, 2008. 14(19): p. 6042-54.

[47] Weissenberger, J, et al., IL-6 is required for glioma development in a mouse model. Oncogene, 2004. 23(19): p. 3308-16.

[48] Doucette, TA, et al., Signal transducer and activator of transcription 3 promotes angiogenesis and drives malignant progression in glioma. Neuro Oncol, 2012.

[49] Sen, M, et al., First-in-Human Trial of a STAT3 Decoy Oligonucleotide in Head and Neck Tumors: Implications for Cancer Therapy. Cancer Discov, 2012. 2(8): p. 694-705.

[50] Gachon, F, et al., The loss of circadian PAR bZip transcription factors results in epilepsy. Genes Dev, 2004. 18(12): p. 1397-412.

[51] Benito, A, et al., A novel role for proline- and acid-rich basic region leucine zipper (PAR bZIP) proteins in the transcriptional regulation of a BH3-only proapoptotic gene. J Biol Chem, 2006. 281(50): p. 38351-7.

[52] De Angelis, R, et al., Functional interaction of the subunit 3 of RNA polymerase II (RPB3) with transcription factor-4 (ATF4). FEBS Lett, 2003. 547(1-3): p. 15-9.

[53] Tian, X, et al., Modulation of CCAAT/enhancer binding protein homologous protein (CHOP)-dependent DR5 expression by nelfinavir sensitizes glioblastoma multiforme cells to tumor necrosis factor-related apoptosis-inducing ligand (TRAIL). J Biol Chem, 2011. 286(33): p. 29408-16.

[54] Blais, JD, et al., Activating transcription factor 4 is translationally regulated by hypoxic stress. Mol Cell Biol, 2004. 24(17): p. 7469-82.

[55] Blank, V and NC Andrews, The Maf transcription factors: regulators of differentiation. Trends Biochem Sci, 1997. 22(11): p. 437-41.

[56] Asting, AG, et al., COX-2 gene expression in colon cancer tissue related to regulating factors and promoter methylation status. BMC Cancer, 2011. 11: p. 238.

[57] Natkunam, Y, et al., Characterization of c-Maf transcription factor in normal and neoplastic hematolymphoid tissue and its relevance in plasma cell neoplasia. Am J Clin Pathol, 2009. 132(3): p. 361-71.

[58] Crawford, EL, et al., CEBPG regulates ERCC5/XPG expression in human bronchial epithelial cells and this regulation is modified by E2F1/YY1 interactions. Carcinogenesis, 2007. 28(12): p. 2552-9.

[59] Mullins, DN, et al., CEBPG transcription factor correlates with antioxidant and DNA repair genes in normal bronchial epithelial cells but not in individuals with bronchogenic carcinoma. BMC Cancer, 2005. 5: p. 141.

[60] O'Donovan, A, et al., Isolation of active recombinant XPG protein, a human DNA repair endonuclease. J Biol Chem, 1994. 269(23): p. 15965-8.

[61] Lee, BK, AA Bhinge, and VR Iyer, Wide-ranging functions of E2F4 in transcriptional activation and repression revealed by genome-wide analysis. Nucleic Acids Res, 2011. 39(9): p. 3558-73.

[62] Graham, JD and CL Clarke, Physiological action of progesterone in target tissues. Endocr Rev, 1997. 18(4): p. 502-19.

[63] Grunberg, SM, et al., Treatment of unresectable meningiomas with the antiprogesterone agent mifepristone. J Neurosurg, 1991. 74(6): p. 861-6.

[64] Schrell, UM, et al., Hormonal dependency of cerebral meningiomas. Part 1: Female sex steroid receptors and their significance as specific markers for adjuvant medical therapy. J Neurosurg, 1990. 73(5): p. 743-9.

[65] Mahesh, VB, DW Brann, and LB Hendry, Diverse modes of action of progesterone and its metabolites. J Steroid Biochem Mol Biol, 1996. 56(1-6 Spec No): p. 209-19.

[66] Tsai, SY and MJ Tsai, Chick ovalbumin upstream promoter-transcription factors (COUP-TFs): coming of age. Endocr Rev, 1997. 18(2): p. 229-40.

[67] Lee, CT, et al., The nuclear orphan receptor COUP-TFII is required for limb and skeletal muscle development. Mol Cell Biol, 2004. 24(24): p. 10835-43.

[68] Takamoto, N, et al., COUP-TFII is essential for radial and anteroposterior patterning of the stomach. Development, 2005. 132(9): p. 2179-89.

[69] You, LR, et al., Suppression of Notch signalling by the COUP-TFII transcription factor regulates vein identity. Nature, 2005. 435(7038): p. 98-104.

[70] You, LR, et al., Mouse lacking COUP-TFII as an animal model of Bochdalek-type congenital diaphragmatic hernia. Proc Natl Acad Sci U S A, 2005. 102(45): p. 16351-6.

[71] Qin, J, et al., COUP-TFII regulates tumor growth and metastasis by modulating tumor angiogenesis. Proc Natl Acad Sci U S A, 2010. 107(8): p. 3687-92.

[72] Shaw, EJ, et al., Gene expression in oligodendroglial tumors. Cell Oncol (Dordr), 2011. 34(4): p. 355-67.

[73] Issemann, I and S Green, Activation of a member of the steroid hormone receptor superfamily by peroxisome proliferators. Nature, 1990. 347(6294): p. 645-50.

[74] Robbins, GT and D Nie, PPAR gamma, bioactive lipids, and cancer progression. Front Biosci, 2012. 17: p. 1816-34.

[75] Cellai, I, et al., Antineoplastic effects of rosiglitazone and PPARgamma transactivation in neuroblastoma cells. Br J Cancer, 2006. 95(7): p. 879-88.

[76] Grommes, C, et al., Inhibition of in vivo glioma growth and invasion by peroxisome proliferator-activated receptor gamma agonist treatment. Mol Pharmacol, 2006. 70(5): p. 1524-33.

[77] Strakova, N, et al., Peroxisome proliferator-activated receptors (PPAR) agonists affect cell viability, apoptosis and expression of cell cycle related proteins in cell lines of glial brain tumors. Neoplasma, 2005. 52(2): p. 126-36.

[78] Chearwae, W and JJ Bright, PPARgamma agonists inhibit growth and expansion of CD133+ brain tumour stem cells. Br J Cancer, 2008. 99(12): p. 2044-53.

[79] Pestereva, E, S Kanakasabai, and JJ Bright, PPARgamma agonists regulate the expression of stemness and differentiation genes in brain tumour stem cells. Br J Cancer, 2012. 106(10): p. 1702-12.

[80] Veliceasa, D, FT Schulze-Hoepfner, and OV Volpert, PPARgamma and Agonists against Cancer: Rational Design of Complementation Treatments. PPAR Res, 2008. 2008: p. 945275.

[81] Oyake, T, et al., Bach proteins belong to a novel family of BTB-basic leucine zipper transcription factors that interact with MafK and regulate transcription through the NF-E2 site. Mol Cell Biol, 1996. 16(11): p. 6083-95.

[82] Shim, KS, et al., Bach2 is involved in neuronal differentiation of N1E-115 neuroblastoma cells. Exp Cell Res, 2006. 312(12): p. 2264-78.

[83] Sasaki, S, et al., Cloning and expression of human B cell-specific transcription factor BACH2 mapped to chromosome 6q15. Oncogene, 2000. 19(33): p. 3739-49.

[84] Hoshino, H, et al., Oxidative stress abolishes leptomycin B-sensitive nuclear export of transcription repressor Bach2 that counteracts activation of Maf recognition element. J Biol Chem, 2000. 275(20): p. 15370-6.

[85] Muto, A, et al., Identification of Bach2 as a B-cell-specific partner for small maf proteins that negatively regulate the immunoglobulin heavy chain gene 3' enhancer. Embo J, 1998. 17(19): p. 5734-43.

[86] Yeung, K, et al., Suppression of Raf-1 kinase activity and MAP kinase signalling by RKIP. Nature, 1999. 401(6749): p. 173-7.

[87] Wu, K and B Bonavida, The activated NF-kappaB-Snail-RKIP circuitry in cancer reg-
      ulates both the metastatic cascade and resistance to apoptosis by cytotoxic drugs.
      Crit Rev Immunol, 2009. 29(3): p. 241-54.

[88] Martinho, O, et al., Downregulation of RKIP is associated with poor outcome and
      malignant progression in gliomas. PLoS ONE, 2012. 7(1): p. e30769.

[89] Ju, W, et al., Identification of genes with differential expression in chemoresistant ep-
      ithelial ovarian cancer using high-density oligonucleotide microarrays. Oncol Res,
      2009. 18(2-3): p. 47-56.

[90] van der Heul-Nieuwenhuijsen, L, NF Dits, and G Jenster, Gene expression of fork-
      head transcription factors in the normal and diseased human prostate. BJU Int, 2009.
      103(11): p. 1574-80.

[91] Pierrou, S, et al., Cloning and characterization of seven human forkhead proteins:
      binding site specificity and DNA bending. Embo J, 1994. 13(20): p. 5002-12.

[92] Smith, KS, et al., Disrupted differentiation and oncogenic transformation of lym-
      phoid progenitors in E2A-HLF transgenic mice. Mol Cell Biol, 1999. 19(6): p. 4443-51.

[93] Shaulian, E and M Karin, AP 1 in cell proliferation and survival. Oncogene, 2001.
      20(19): p. 2390-400.

[94] Schreiber, M, et al., Control of cell cycle progression by c-Jun is p53 dependent.
      Genes Dev, 1999. 13(5): p. 607-19.

[95] Wilson, RE, et al., Early response gene signalling cascades activated by ionising radi-
      ation in primary human B cells. Oncogene, 1993. 8(12): p. 3229-37.

[96] Liu, Y, et al., Inhibition of AP-1 transcription factor causes blockade of multiple sig-
      nal transduction pathways and inhibits breast cancer growth. Oncogene, 2002. 21(50):
      p. 7680-9.

[97] Libermann, TA and LF Zerbini, Targeting transcription factors for cancer gene thera-
      py. Curr Gene Ther, 2006. 6(1): p. 17-33.

[98] Wieser, R, The oncogene and developmental regulator EVI1: expression, biochemical
      properties, and biological functions. Gene, 2007. 396(2): p. 346-57.

[99] Koos, B, et al., The transcription factor evi-1 is overexpressed, promotes proliferation,
      and is prognostically unfavorable in infratentorial ependymomas. Clin Cancer Res,
      2011. 17(11): p. 3631-7.

[100] Zardo, G, et al., Integrated genomic and epigenomic analyses pinpoint biallelic gene
      inactivation in tumors. Nat Genet, 2002. 32(3): p. 453-8.

[101] Zhao, LY, et al., An EBF3-mediated transcriptional program that induces cell cycle
      arrest and apoptosis. Cancer Res, 2006. 66(19): p. 9445-52.

[102] Liao, D, Emerging roles of the EBF family of transcription factors in tumor suppres-
      sion. Mol Cancer Res, 2009. 7(12): p. 1893-901.

[103] Wang, H, et al., C/EBPalpha arrests cell proliferation through direct inhibition of Cdk2 and Cdk4. Mol Cell, 2001. 8(4): p. 817-28.

[104] Pabst, T, et al., Dominant-negative mutations of CEBPA, encoding CCAAT/enhancer binding protein-alpha (C/EBPalpha), in acute myeloid leukemia. Nat Genet, 2001. 27(3): p. 263-70.

[105] Yoon, K and RC Smart, C/EBPalpha is a DNA damage-inducible p53-regulated mediator of the G1 checkpoint in keratinocytes. Mol Cell Biol, 2004. 24(24): p. 10650-60.

[106] Thompson, EA, et al., C/EBPalpha expression is downregulated in human nonmelanoma skin cancers and inactivation of C/EBPalpha confers susceptibility to UVB-induced skin squamous cell carcinomas. J Invest Dermatol, 2011. 131(6): p. 1339-46.

[107] Ravanpay, AC and JM Olson, E protein dosage influences brain development more than family member identity. J Neurosci Res, 2008. 86(7): p. 1472-81.

[108] Uittenbogaard, M and A Chiaramello, Expression of the bHLH transcription factor Tcf12 (ME1) gene is linked to the expansion of precursor cell populations during neurogenesis. Brain Res Gene Expr Patterns, 2002. 1(2): p. 115-21.

[109] O'Neil, J, et al., TAL1/SCL induces leukemia by inhibiting the transcriptional activity of E47/HEB. Cancer Cell, 2004. 5(6): p. 587-96.

[110] Riemenschneider, MJ, TH Koy, and G Reifenberger, Expression of oligodendrocyte lineage genes in oligodendroglial and astrocytic gliomas. Acta Neuropathol, 2004. 107(3): p. 277-82.

[111] Shu, HK, et al., The intrinsic radioresistance of glioblastoma-derived cell lines is associated with a failure of p53 to induce p21(BAX) expression. Proc Natl Acad Sci U S A, 1998. 95(24): p. 14453-8.

[112] Rubel, A, et al., The membrane targeted apoptosis modulators erucylphosphocholine and erucylphosphohomocholine increase the radiation response of human glioblastoma cell lines in vitro. Radiat Oncol, 2006. 1: p. 6.

[113] Honda, N, et al., Radiosensitization by overexpression of the nonphosphorylation form of IkappaB-alpha in human glioma cells. J Radiat Res, 2002. 43(3): p. 283-92.

[114] Yamagishi, N, J Miyakoshi, and H Takebe, Enhanced radiosensitivity by inhibition of nuclear factor kappa B activation in human malignant glioma cells. Int J Radiat Biol, 1997. 72(2): p. 157-62.

[115] Struhl, K, Gene regulation. A paradigm for precision. Science, 2001. 293(5532): p. 1054-5.

[116] Chen, X, et al., Integration of external signaling pathways with the core transcriptional network in embryonic stem cells

Stem Cells

Chapter 8

Brain Tumor Stemness

Andrés Felipe Cardona and León Darío Ortíz

Additional information is available at the end of the chapter

1. Introduction

The incidence of primary tumors of the central nervous system (CNS) has been estimated in 15.8/100,000 and 17.2/100,000 individuals for men and women, respectively [1,2], which globally represents approximately 190,000 new cases per year. They represent the 3rd most common cause of death from cancer in middle-aged men, and the 4th most common in women between 15 and 34 years of age [3,4]. The most frequent tumors called gliomas exhibit glial characteristics on pathologic examination [1,3]. Despite advances in the knowledge of the molecular biology of gliomas, effective therapeutic strategies remain elusive. After multimodality treatment with surgery, radiation and chemotherapy, the overall survival (OS) of patients with Glioblastoma (GB), the most frequent glioma, is around 14.6 months and the survival at 2 years is 26% [5, 6, 7, 8]. Although it is recognized that there are progenitor cells that can differentiate into neuronal and glial cells, the concept of a brain tumor stem cells is more controversial. In 2002, Altman and colleagues proposed the theory of post-natal neurogenesis that, associated with the finding of progenitor cells in glial tumors, suggested that these cells could be targeted for more effective therapies[9]. One of the difficulties is that there are no specific phenotypic markers for these cancer stem cells, and, therefore, their identification is limited to a functional characterization.

Nonetheless, pluripotent cells obtained from human brain tumors that express the CD133 surface marker (or Prominin 1; PROM1 is the founding member of pentaspantransmembrane glycoproteins) have the ability for sustained self-renewal, proliferation and tumor initiation/propagation. Furthermore, this functionally defined glioma stem cells form a niche around the blood vessels, being highly pro- angiogenic; those are regulated by hypoxia and are resistant to conventional oncologic treatment like radiotherapy and/or chemotherapy [10, 11]. In addition, they have important migration and invasion capabilities while actively interacting with the immune system. Therefore, therapeutic opportunities include targeting of stem cell specific pathways, induction of differentiation of stem cells, blocking microenvironment signals (including angiogenesis factors), and harnessing the immune system to recognize and attack stem cells. Significant challenges continues since the presence of cancer stem cells within the tumor is highly heterogenous, they can remain quiescent for years, and they may share biological features with normal stem cells [12, 13].

We present here a detailed review of the published literature on cancer stem cells of gliomas and meduloblastomas, and their possible relationships with the response to chemo-radio-therapy and to future therapeutic interventions. Similarly, we discuss their role in the progression of the disease, and we provide an analysis of the functional properties of neuronal progenitor cells and of their tumor homologues that lose their regulatory capacity during the process of neurogenesis.

2. Identification of progenitor cells in the brain and the relationship with glial tumors

Cancer only develops after mutations occurs in a few cells. These abnormal cells lose the capacity for self -regulation and have the potential for uncontrolled proliferation [12]. Two hypothetical models have been invoked to explain this phenomenon. The first is the "stochastic" which predicts that all cells have a homogeneous capacity to initiate a neoplasm with areas in which the elements are activated in a synchronic and constitutive manner [12]. The second model is the "hierarchic" which assumes that only a sub-group of cells in the tumor has the potential to proliferate and to generate new neoplasic focus; the other cells act as support or represent well-differentiated or terminal tumor cells. This model explains the findings of the pluripotent progenitor cells in acute myeloid leukemia, in cerebral tumors, and in cancer of the breast, prostate and colon [13, 14]. Nevertheless, those two models are not exclusive and it is likely that there is a combination of both scenarios in most types of cancer. Fig. (1) Summarizes the principal molecular alterations of cerebral tumors of glial origin.

Early studies by Nottebohm et al. reported the discovery of neural embryonic tissue in the cerebral parenchyma of birds [15],followed by reports of similar findings in rodents, primates and humans [16]. As a consequence, it is generally accepted that neurogenesis persists during adulthood, particularly at the level of the dentate gyrus of the hippocampus (in the hilus and in several planes of the granular laminae) and in the upper region of the deep lateral ventricles, neighboring the striated body, as shown in Fig. (2).These cells constitute about 0.2% of the elements forming the encephalon, primitively associated with the telencephalon and generally expressing the glial fibrillary acidic protein (GFAP) [16, 17]. They have a putative role in, and are capable of regenerating the neurogenetic structure in vivo and in vitro; generally enjoying a state of relative quiescence with a cell cycle of about 28 days (type B cells or pluripotent astrocytes) [18].

Usually, the pluripotent progenitor cells have a capacity of generating other second-order progenitor elements that divide every 12 hours (rapid proliferation phase). These cells, termed type C (immature precursors), maintain multipotent capacity and generate other neuronal precursors with greater maturity, termed type A cells (migrant neuroblasts). This type A cells are capable of migrating in groups across the rostral portion of the lateral ventricle up to the olfactory bulb where they are integrated as new interneurons in different layers of the cortex (Fig. 2) [19].The subventricular stem cells are conserved in eutherian mammals, but only in man is the cellular displacement not grouped, but rather individual; and follow a destiny that, as-yet, has not been clarified [20]. Analogously to the subventricular zone, the hippocampus granular region amplifies some lesser-known precursor cells termed type D, which have limited migratory capacity (short distances) [20].

From the neurochemical perspective, the type B cells express intermediate filaments such as vimentin and nestin, and are characteristically negative for the neuronal markers PSA-NCAM (Poly-Sialated Neural Cell Adhesion Molecule) and TuJ1 (class III beta-tubulin) [21]. They frequently express PDGFR-α (platelet-derived growth factor receptor) which appears to act as a regulator of balance for the differentiation between the oligodendrocytes and neurons during the phase of asymmetric neurogenesis. The type B cells, while being highly sensitive to stimulation by epidermal growth factor (EGF) and FGF2 (fibroblast growth factor type 2) [20], show constitutive positivity for CD133.

The expression of CD133 marker has been observed in normal progenitor cells, glial tumors and central nervous system neoplasms ("neurosphere" model) [22, 23]. CD133 is a 130 KDa surface glycoprotein with 5 transmembrane domains [24]. There are several isoforms of CD133 regulated by methylation, but their specific regulatory roles in transcription are still unknown [24]. Some reports suggest that their position in the membrane has some relationship with the dynamic organization of cell structure and, as such, determines cell polarity, migration and interaction with other neighboring cells, especially with those belonging to the tumor endothelium [21, 25]. The CD133 positive (CD133+) cells have a series of mechanisms that contribute to preferential activation of regulatory points of the cell cycle, increasing its resistance to standard chemotherapy and radiation therapy. [26]. This finding and other routes of abnormal activation such as Wnt/β-catenin (Wnt was coined as a combination of Wg and Int and can be pronounced as 'wint'), Notch (The notch signaling pathway is a highly conserved cell signaling system present in most multicellular organism), SHh (sonic-hedgehog), PTEN (phosphatase and tensin homolog) and Bmi-1 (polycomb ring finger oncogene) explain, at least in part, why progenitor cells of glial tumors are resistant to radiotherapy [26, 27]. In addition, these cells exhibit primary resistance to chemotherapy agents like carboplatin, paclitaxel and etoposide [28, 29].

GB are remarkably heterogeneous tumors, both phenotypically and genetically, and it is very unlikely that a single antigen will selectively identify a single population of uniquely tumorigenic cells that is common to all GBs. It is important to note that CD133-negative brain tumor cells can also generate tumors in murine cancer models, and those new cells can express CD133 in celular membrane [30]. In human tissue, another investigation have shown that A2B5, a glial progenitor marker, is expressed in human gliomas, up to 61.7% of tumoral cells, viewed on flow cytometry [31]. It would be considered that the role of CD133+ cells, versus the rest of the cell population, in brain tumor initiation and progression is still uncertain, but most of studies and models agree with the importance of CD133+ cells in tumorgenesis on the brain [16-29].

A study that evaluated the genetic expression of the BCRP1/ABCG2 (also known as Abcg2 murine/ABCG2 human) and MGMT (O-6-methylguanine-DNA methyltransferase) in glial progenitors found a significant increase in their activity, similar to various apoptosis suppressors such as Bcl-2 (B-cell lymphoma 2, apoptosis checkpoint), FLIP (inhibitory protein), BCL-XL ("B-cell lymphoma-extra large", involved in the signal transduction pathway of the FAS-L.) and of some inhibitors of pro-apoptosis proteins such as XIAP (Co-chaperone of The hsp90, immunophilin homolog XAP2), cIAP1 (cellular inhibitor of apoptosis 1), cIAP2 (cellular inhibitor of apoptosis 2), NAIP (neuronal apoptosis inhibitory protein) and survivin (baculoviral inhibitor of apoptosis repeat-containing 5 or BIRC5) [23]. Furthermore, the inhibition of the caspases 3, 7 and 9 is significantly higher in recurrent GB rich in CD133+ cells than in its counterpart in which lower counts are observed [32].

Nestin, an intermediate class IV filament that is produced in considerable quantities in normal and tumor progenitor cells during brain development and in glial neoplasms [33, 34], is a constituent part of the cytoskeleton, has the responsibility for the maintenance of the cell morphology and facilitates adhesion, proliferation and migration. In adults, nestin is expressed in the subventricular progenitor cells, in some remnants near the choroid plexus and in the prosencephalon [35]. As in high grade gliomas, nestin is re-expressed in multiple cell lines of the brain during other circumstances such as acute ischemia, trauma and meningo-encephalitis [36]. In neoplasms, the co-expression of nestin and vimentin is related to substantial increase in invasive capacity (associated with multifocality), the facility to repair external attack (nuclear nestin regulates chromatin), and motility. This combination of markers could be useful in assessing the prognosis, especially since its presence is associated to a more aggressive tumor phenotype, rich in progenitor cells [37].

The normal and tumor precursor cells share the expression of multiple markers, the capacity of unlimited regeneration, exponential proliferation and open differentiation. Additionally, they have similar telomerase activity and resistance to apoptosis, as well as a higher capacity to transport substances to membrane level [38]. The latter characteristic facilitates the exocyte of anti-neoplastic molecules via proteins of the ABC family, such as MDR-1 (Gene that encodes P-glycoprotein; ABCB1, ATP-binding cassette, sub-family B member 1), MRP-1 (human multidrug resistance protein or ABCC1), ABCA2, ABCA3 and ABCG2 (Genes that encodes the ATP-binding cassette sub-family A member 2 protein, sub-family A member 3 protein and sub-family G member 2 protein; respectively) [21, 38, 39].

3. Molecular changes that favor tumor progenitor cells

The progenitor cells of brain tumors have certain characteristics that differentiate them from their normal counterparts. By definition, the cancer stem cells need to have the capacity to develop tumors following orthotopic implantation (if the tumor is an identical phenotypic copy of the original tumor). They exhibit a sustained capacity for self-renewal and are capable of showing polyclonality [33]. Reilly et al. established a murine model that combined mutations in the p53 gene and in the gene specific for neurofibromatosis (Nf1, neurofibromin 11), capable of activating the Ras (a protein superfamily of small GTPases) pathway to favor the formation of astrocytomas. They found that the deletion of any tumor suppressor gene and/or the activation of oncogenes such as Ras and Akt (serine/threonine protein kinase) in the undifferentiated cells that express CD133 or nestin, resulted in the formation of glial tumors [40].

Another important alteration is view on PDGF. The effect of PDGF on the nestin-positive progenitor cells is equivalent to that which occurs when the loss of CDKN2A (cyclin-dependent kinase inhibitor 2A), which codes for the INK4a (tumour suppressor protein) and ARF (ADP-ribosylation factor 11) is combined with the increase in the expression of EGFR in the immature and in the mature cells [36,41]. Further, during embryogenesis neural progenitors have been shown to express the A isoform of the PDGFR, while its mature homologue (glia and neurons) is expressed on the PDGF surface. PDGFR-B is found in small quantities in pluriultipotent cells, but only increases as the cells differentiate and mature, especially into oligodendrocytes, and in the presence of phosphorylated PDGFR-A [42]. Infusion of PDGF-A in the subventricular region of certain rodents suppresses the production of neuroblasts and generates a hyperplasia of type B cells which frequently results in the development of astrocytomas and oligodendrogliomas. Additionally, activation, via the PDGF signaling, in the regions of the brain rich in precursor cells contributes to tumorigenesis, which seems to be favored by autocrine and paracrine stimulation of PDGF-A, PDGF-B and the OLIG2 (oligodendrocyte lineage transcription factor 2) transcription factors [42, 43].

Some of the signaling pathways included in the evolution of progenitor cells and in their differentiation are altered in the gliomas. The Notch pathway is essential for the maintenance of tumor cell architecture. It is expressed from embryogenesis and interacts, normally or abnormally, with multiple ligands such as DLL-1, 3 and 4 (delta-like 1, 3 and 4 respectively), together with the Jag-1 and Jag-2 proteins (jagged 1 and 2 respectively). The Notch signaling pathway controls neural differentiation and is known to maintain CNS character and to inhibit neurogenesis. The Notch–Hes (Hairy and enhancer of split) pathway is necessary for self-renewing cell division and, thus, maintenance of the neural precursor population [44-47]. Another recent studies have shown that Fbw7 acts as a molecular switch that antagonizes Notch activity and JNK/c-Jun signaling to enable neural stem cell differentiation and progenitor survival [48]. In tumor progenitors, the Notch receptors has been shown acting as a trigger for stimulation of differentiation [49] and, in preclinical studies, it has been shown experimental therapeutic implications [50]. Differentiation is mediated by tumor necrosis factor- α (TNF-α) activator enzyme and by the C-secretase, which is responsible for the signal transcription to the nucleus for unlinking responses via transcription factor CBF1/Su(H)/LAG1 (CSL) (homologous Drosophila gene Suppressor of Hairless /Longevity assurance gene 1 or cardiolipinsynthetase) [49]. This interaction results in the activation of target genes responsible for preempting differentiation and apoptosis [49] and gives the opportunity for developing therapeutic options [49, 50]. The Notch signaling pathway prevents the degradation and ubiquitous distribution of nestin in the progenitor cells, and cooperates with K-Ras (v-Ki-ras2; Kirsten rat sarcoma viral oncogene homolog) in promoting colony formation [49-51].

A study demonstrated that the inhibition of the Notch-1 receptor induces apoptosis and inhibits the proliferation of glial cell tumors that express CD133 [52]. This provides an opportunity to modulate the pathways responsible of treatment resistance, since there are compounds available that act as decoys, as inhibitors of ϒ-secretase, as intracellular bait directed against MAML-1 (mastermind-like 1), or simply as inhibitors of the Ras pathway [53, 54].

Epithelial Growth Factor is another important issue in the molecular changes on progenitor cells. Using the model of the neurosphere [22], Singh et al. inoculated cells isolated from high grade glioma into the cranium of immuno-suppressed rodents and observed that the minimum number of cells required to produce a neoplasm was 1x105. However, when the experiment was repeated using CD133+ cells stimulated by EGF, the number required was reduced to 100-fold [25, 55]. It is important to note that CD133 expression occurs not only in the neural and neoplastic progenitor cells but also in endothelial stem cells that participate in blood vessel formation necessary for the development of normal brain and for tumorigenesis [55, 56]. In preclinical models, activated EGFR signaling induce behaviors characteristic of GB on stem cells, including enhanced proliferation, survival and migration, even in the absence of EGF ligand. wtEGFR block neuronal differentiation and is associated with a dramatic increase in chemotaxis in the presence of EGF. EGFRvIII expression lead to an increase in neural stem cells proliferation and survival, while it simultaneously blocked neuronal differentiation and promoted glial fate. It gives an opportunity for terapeutic development on this EGF field [57].

4. The micro-environment of progenitor cells and glial tumors

The presence of progenitor cells in Acute Myeloid Leukemia highlights the importance of the micro-environment in maintaining its function, and the quiescent state [9, 12, 14]. The perivascular niche of the glial tumor progenitor cells is highly specialized and depends, in great part, on the capillaries that are similar to those in the periventricular region of the human brain. At the proximity to the endothelial cells, enables inter-cellular communication that causes enrichment with brain derived neurotrophic factor (BDNF), vascular endothelial growth factor C (VEGF-C) and pigment factor derived from the endothelium (PEDF) [9]; molecules that facilitate, principally, migration and neoplasic proliferation. Even more, there is consistent evidence that the extra-cellular matrix is responsible for key points in the regulation of tumor precursors via the tenascin-C gene. Expression of this gene by the cells of the neural crest translates into anti-adhesive properties that block the interaction of fibronectin with the syndecans [58]. Further, chondroitin sulfate continues stimulating the progenitor cell to maintain its primitive state, and impedes evolution of its progeny.

Although the niche affects the biology of the progenitor cells in the tumor, the communication is not unidirectional. Several studies have demonstrated that the precursors are able to promote the replication of endothelial cells, including the necessary stimulus for the formation of complex neovascular structures [59, 60] by increasing the concentrations of VEGF and BDNF [9, 60, 61]. Complementing these data, Calabrese et al. found, using multi-photon laser scanning microscopy, that the CD133+/nestin+ cells were always found in the intimal layer proximal to the vascular endothelium of GB, medulloblastomas, ependymomas and oligodendrogliomas [61].

Classically, pathology of high-grade gliomas describes a disorganized and aberrant vascular growth randomly generated to supply the voracity of the tumor. However, several recently published reviews explain that this architecture is available in the altered form to serve as lodging for the tumor precursors and their vascular analogues [9, 14].

Glial progenitor cells and their descendants are capable of interfering with the blood vessels of the brain, using the effect known as "perivascular satellitosis". Nevertheless, it is infrequent to find extra-axial lesions. Clinically, the microvascular density of GB correlates with prognosis [62]; a factor that contributes to the response observed in anti-angiogenesis, possibly dependent on VEGF generated in elevated quantities by the CD133+ cells [63, 64]. Further, the observation that CD133+ GB cells lose their ability to recruit endothelial cells and form blood vessels after being exposed to low concentrations of bevacizumab suggests that this effect is controlled, at least in part, by the decrease in the expression of VEGF, VEGFR2 and angiopoietin-2 (Ang-2) [9].

Data from pre-clinical studies and clinical trials indicate that three drugs that block angiogenesis may be promising therapy for high-grade gliomas, due to their inhibitory potential on the niche of tumor progenitors. An estudy demonstrated that endothelial cells increase brain tumor stem cell survival and targeting the tumor vasculature with bevacizumab reduces the number of cancer stem cells in treated tumors [65]. Bevacizumab (humanized monoclonal antibody against VEGF receptors 1 and 2) and cediranib (AZD2171, potent inhibitor of VEGF receptor tyrosine kinases type 1, 2 and 3) are being evaluated currently in clinical trials. [65, 66, 67]Those are agents that act on the VEGF 1, 2 and 3 receptors, suggesting an improvement in progression- free survival (PFS) and OS in patients with recurrent high grade gliomas. Cilengitide blocks the $\alpha v\beta 6$, $\alpha v\beta 5$ y $\alpha v\beta 3$ integrins [68] and has been evaluated in clinical trials [69, 70]. As previously mentioned, the effect of these molecules is the normalization of the tumor vessels, or the depletion of the blood flow, that interferes with the maintenance and survival of the precursor and terminal cells of the tumor, thus, anti-angiogenic therapy may function as a therapy against Glioma Stem Cells. A further nuance has come from early studies that suggest that glioblastoma cells can form parts of the tumor vasculature [71]. It is likely that anti-angiogenic drugs might not only inhibit tumor vascularization to suppress GB growth, but also directly disrupt the niches for the maintenance of GSCs, therefore weakening the "tumor roots".

5. Role of progenitor cells in meduloblastomas

The two germinal epithelia of the cerebellum are found in the deep ventricular zone of the velum of the posterior medulla and in the outermost layer of the metencephalon [72]. The matrix of the first of these regions gives rise to several neuronal and glial cell lines, and the second, only produces granular cells which are the most numerous elements in all of the prosencephalon [73]. In humans, peak growth of the cerebellum occurs later in comparison with the remainder of the CNS, and its principal stage of development is in the third trimester of gestation. In other more rudimentary mammalians this event occurs during the two weeks following birth [74]. Nevertheless, evolution of this neural structure is observed in children up to the end of the first year of life, and appears to be dependent on the presence of the CD133+ cells, which are concentrated principally in the white matter and in the rhombic lips [75].

The evidence that connects the pluripotent neural cells with the tumor elements of the meduloblastoma is merely correlative and is supported by the expression of the calbindin-D (calcium binding protein D) among the precursors of normal cerebellum and, as well as being found in 50% of the meduloblastomas, especially in those of the classical type. In contrast, nodular lesions or desmoplasias express the marker p75, which suggests a dual tumor origin. This hypothesis is supported by the behavior of the meduloblastomas induced in murine models that frequently express CD133+ but which have a specific dissimilar evolution such as, among other aspects, the aberrant activation of the Hedgehog (Hh) gene [76].

The Hh pathway regulates the development of the cerebellum in many species, but has cardinal importance among humans, where it promotes migration of precursors of granular cells, and their proliferation incited by the production of the Hh ligand in Purkinje cells. The mutation in the PTCH (patched homolog 1) receptor which results in constitutive activation of the Hh pathway is found in a great number of patients with sporadic meduloblastoma, as well as in those with Gorlin syndrome, an autosomal dominant entity characterized by coexistence of basal cell carcinomas and primitive neuroectodermal tumors [73, 75]. Approximately 14% of the mice heterozygous for the PTCH mutation develop medulobastomas, in which primary alterations of the precursors of the granular cells are frequently found, as well as changes in the SMO (smoothened) and SUFU (suppressor of fused homolog) genes, which are generators of this type of neoplasia in vivo [77]. Other animal models have demonstrated that meduloblastomas initiated by genetic changes in the different pathways of Hh also result in the activation of this signaling pathway; in particular, the inactivation of the CXCR6 (chemokine receptor CXCR6) that results in the expression of Gli1, Gli2 (GLI family zinc finger 1 and 2), Ptc2 (Hh receptor Patched type 2) and Sfrp1(secreted frizzled-related protein 1) proteins evident in the meduloblastomas, and which are susceptible to inhibition of Hh with molecules such as cyclopamine, or with specific inhibitors such as Hh-antagonist [78].

Another signaling pathway altered in sporadic and inherited meduloblastomas is the Wingless/Wnt (wingless-type MMTV integration site family member) that regulates the proliferation of progenitor cells in the deep ventricular region and in the hippocampus [9]. The loss of Wnt1, a key effector of β-catenin, causes several abnormalities in the midbrain and in the cerebellum, and is found over-expressed in classical meduloblastomas [79, 80]. Although its role in the regulation of the pluripotent progenitors of the cerebellum is not clear, it appears to depend on similar mutations to those identified in the patients with Turcot syndrome; an autosomal recessive condition caused by the loss of function of the adenomatous polyposis gene, and which is present in 5% of medulloblastomas [80]. The mutations have also been observed in a small subgroup of patients with primitive neuroectoderm tumors and results in the decrease in expression of Axin-2 (plays an important role in the regulation of the stability of beta-catenin in the Wnt signaling pathway); the gene that acts as negative regulator of Wnt and which has been detected in a small group of patients with medulloblastoma [81].

The nuclear translocation of the β-catenin resulting in the activation of the Wnt pathway is observed in 25% of the patients with medulloblastoma and, usually, corresponds to an elevated presence of the CD133 cells. Paradoxically, and in contrary to what occurs in high-grade gliomas, their presence is associated with a favorable clinical evolution, related to the absence of alterations in Hh and aberrations in chromosome 17 [82].

The Notch signaling pathway is observed to be active in the progenitor cells of the deep ventricular region and in the rhombic region. It promotes proliferation and survival and inhibits cellular differentiation. The four isoforms of the receptor do not result in the same changes in the cerebellum. For example, Notch-2 stimulates the proliferation of progenitors of the granular neuromas, while Notch-1 is associated with their differentiation; a consistent finding in the classical forms of medulloblastomas [82]. Some primitive neuroectoderm tumors show increase in the Notch-2 loci and in co-expression of the Hes1 pathway, that correlate clinically with adverse prognosis; while other studies have provided evidence for alternative and abnormal regulation Notch Hh pathway [72]. Finally, hypoxia and the protein products that this activity generates, promote the proliferation of progenitor cells of the cerebellum stimulated by the Notch pathway; a finding that has been confirmed in medulloblastomas [83]. Fig. (3) summarizes the principal signaling pathways of the neural precursors of the cerebellum and of medulloblastomas.

Several subordinate pathways can promote the generation of medulloblastomas from neural progenitor cells. The REN (renin) gene located on chromosome 17 promotes the differentiation of granular precursors, suppressing the Hh signals, an alteration that frequently results in medulloblastoma [73]. The N-myc oncogene (v-mycmyelocytomatosis viral related oncogene, neuroblastoma derived), which plays an essential role in cerebellum growth, is a primary constituent of white matter of the Hh pathway in medulloblastoma and is observed to be amplified in large cell variants, which favor a negative clinical outcome. Other transcription factors associated with the more primitive processes of progenitor cells of the cerebellum and tumor development are RE-1 (RE1-Silencing Transcription factor), OTX2 (orthodenticle homolog 2) and BMI1 (BMI1 polycomb ring finger oncogene) [72, 73]. A recent report described the substantial role of molecular alterations of CD15+/CD133– in the induction of primitive neuroectoderm brain tumors [84].

6. Therapeutic implications of tumor progenitors

The prognostic implications of the presence of stem cells in gliomas has been examined in a few clinical trials. A study that included 44 patients with GB treated surgically followed by radiotherapy and temozolamide (TMZ), evaluated the prognostic value of CD133 expression and of the capacity of the tumor to generate CD133+ cells in culture. The CD133 status, as determined by immunohistochemistry, had no prognostic value, but the in vitro capacity to generate precursors was associated to a significant reduction in OS (HR: 2.50; 95%CI: 1.04-6.06; P = 0.004) of 8 (95%CI: 4.0-11.5) and 15 months (95%CI: 11.0-19.0) for tumors with higher and lower quantity of CD133+ cells, respectively (P = 0.0002). Similarly, the PFS was also associated to the ability to generate precursors from the tumor (3.5 months for high versus 9.0 months for low grade; P = 0.0001). The CD133+ count was also associated with a higher mortality risk (HR: 1.65; 95%CI: 1.05-2.60; P = 0.0285) [85]. A similar study examining high grade oligodendrogliomas found that tumors without CD133+ cells had an improved prognosis, and this marker predicted clinical outcome better than histological assessment [86]. Another immunohistochemical analysis for nestin and CD133 of both, low grade and high grade gliomas, revealed that their expression correlates with survival, with tumors that co-express nestin+/CD133+ carrying a shorter survival [87]. These findings have stimulated the active search for new therapeutic strategies directed against the precursors of cerebral tumors, and their microenvironment.

Therapeutic interventions directed against cerebral tumor progenitor cells can be divided into three groups: firstly, directed towards provoking differentiation of the precursors; secondly, designed to eliminate the progenitor cells inhibiting their multi-potentiality and quiescence; thirdly, directed towards attacking the tumor microenvironment [88, 89].

The therapies that provoke differentiation of the progenitors focus on the capacity to reverse the malignant state and, essentially, to recover the auto-regenerative property [90]. To-date, two groups of medications affect differentiation: derivatives of retinoic acid and compounds directed against epigenetic changes (histone deacetylators).

Among the compounds directed towards eliminating progenitor cells, the therapies of note are those that are directed against tumor markers of progenitor cells expressed in cellular membrane (antibodies against CD133+) [9], the inhibitors of the Hh pathway (cyclopamine, NBT-272) [91], PPAR-γ agonists [92], TMZ [93], inhibitors of mTOR (sirolimus, everolimus, temsirolimus, deforolimus) [94], derivatives of bone morphogenetic protein (BMP) [95], target molecules directed against check-points that avoid damage induced by radiotherapy in the progenitors (Chk1 and Chk2, checkpoint homolog type 1 and 2) [15], imatinib [96, 97] and inhibitors of the ABCB super-family [98]. Similarly, it is important to mention the drugs that modify the micro-environment, among which are the angiogenesis blocking drugs such as bevacizumab [65], cediranib [67] and cilengitide [68, 69] and, equally, the inhibitors of PI3K (phosphoinositide-3-kinase) that could act turning the medulloblastoma progenitors closest to the vascular niche more sensitive to irradiation, as in vitro studies show for human endothelial cells precursors [99]. Fig. (4) highlights some strategies directed against the cell precursors of brain tumors.

The effect of retinoic acid on the CD133+ cells appears to be related to the repression of the Wnt/β-catenin pathway that slows the proliferation accompanying over-expression of Axin [100]. The same strategy is used in a preclinical model to test the effectiveness of combining 13-cis-retenoic acid with vorinostat (SAHA) in medulloblastoma cells in culture. Retinoic acid acts on the transcriptional activation of BMP-2 (Bone morphogenetic protein 2), and SA-HA facilitates the apopotosis controlling chromatin; effects that lead to an increase in the sensitivity to cisplatin and etoposide [101]. Heat shock protein 90 (HSP90) operates as a supplier of β-catenin during its conformational maturation phase. The inhibitor 17-allylamino-17-demethoxygeldanamycin (17-AAG) modifies the HSP90 phenotype and affects the aberrant expression of the β-catenin. This enables the inhibition (in vivo and in vitro) of the growth of several cell lines of glioma and their progenitors CD133+, and translates into an increase in the effect of radiation on the GB; a finding that is more evident during exposure to TMZ [102].

With respect to the preponderant role of Hh in the development of normal and tumor progenitor cells, Bar et al explored the effectiveness of cyclopamine in a subpopulation of primordial GB cells [103]. In the study, 26% of the samples showed Gli (transcription factors mediating the Hh pathway isolated from Glioblastoma) over-expression, a target function of this pathway that was inhibited satisfactorily in 60% of the cases. The outcome was a significant decrease in the CD133+ progenitor growth. In parallel, the administration of cyclopamine on neurospheres inhibited the generation of new colonies, suggesting a regression of the clonogenic capacity of the glioma progenitors.

Beier et al. demonstrated that TMZ is incapable of inducing death of the CD133+ cells. Proliferation was effectively inhibited by reducing its metabolism in vitro by 72% following 7 days of incubation [93]. Depending on the subtype of cells, TMZ induces arrest in the G2-M transition or delay in the cell cycle at G2. However, in all the cultures, the cells at sub-G0 peak of apoptosis, was <8%. Genetical analysis shows that the pattern of presentation of the promoter of the MGMT gene was greater among the negative cells, which does not explain the susceptibility of the progenitors to the alkylating agent [93].

Glial progenitors and their progeny conserve a mechanism of homogeneous differentiation promoted by BMP (bone morphogenetic protein) and its ligands, reducing slightly the quantity of CD133+ cells and favoring the increase in the astroglia and of the cellular elements, similar to neurons. An study observed in some in vivo models that the therapeutic stimulus of the different isoforms of BMP delays tumor growth and the potential for vascular invasion of the GB [104].

Cancer stem cells from GB specimens seems to be immune suppressive as they inhibit mitogen T cell proliferation from normal donors [105].Therefore targeting specifically cancer stem cells may revert the immune suppressive microenvironment induced by these cells, allowing a synergistic effect when combined with immune therapy. On the other hand GB derived stem cells may be a source of unique antigens that can be used for dendritic cell vaccination, as has been demonstrated in the animal model [106].

As previously mentioned, the use of bevacizumab attenuates the capacity of the tumor progenitors to promote angiogenesis, and it will be seen not only following the regulation of acidosis and hypoxia but also by the activation of oncogenes such as PTEN and EGFR [64, 107]. Cediranib, a pan-inhibitor of VEGF receptor, normalizes the blood vessels of the tumor in patients with recurrent GB; the perilesional edema is alleviated and the capacity for pre-production of the CD133+ progenitors and the endothelium precursor cells is reduced [66]. Cilengitide reduces the expression of $\alpha v \beta 3$ integrin in the tumor micro-environment. The migratory and proliferative capacity of the precursors is reduced by up to 60%; an effect that appears to be dependent on the dose and on the co-expression of other surface antigens of the endothelial cells (CD144 and von Willebrand factor) [68-70].

Aldehyde dehydrogenase function is used by cancer stem cells to repopulate a tumor mass after chemotherapy cytoreduction. As in hematopoyetic stem cells, it would be spected that inhibition of Aldehyde dehydrogenase helps differentiate cells. With the inhibition of aldehyde dehydrogenase, stem cell division to non-stem daughter cells tends to become blocked. Exist potent aldehyde dehydrogenase inhibitors on the market: chloral hydrate, chloramphenicol, and disulfiram, that could be useful [108].

7. Conclusion

Our understanding about cancer and the relationship with the theory of stem cells is growing up as the tumoral incidence around the world does.

Advances in molecular cell biology will give to the oncology physicians and scientist the tools for understanding the processes underlying tumorgenesis and intracelullar processes for viability, serving as possible targets in oncotherapy, diagnosis and prognosis.

Molecular characteristics that give susceptibility for brain tumors to some therapies encourage the clinicians to become experts for giving the best therapeutic choices according to molecular guidance for radio/chemotherapy or other alternatives, like biological therapy, immunotherapy and experimental treatment options.

Future about stem cells as a chapter of brain tumors is on the road for establish individualized treatment profiles, depending on clinical, pathological and molecular characteristics of patients and tumors, a traslational analysis from the molecules to the patients.

Author details

Andrés Felipe Cardona[1,2*] and León Darío Ortíz[2,3]

*Address all correspondence to: a_cardonaz@yahoo.com andres.cardona@fsfb.org.co

1 Clinical and Translational Oncology Group, Institute of Oncology, Fundación Santa Fe de Bogotá, Bogotá D.C., Colombia

2 Red LANO/ONCOL Group, Colombia

3 Neuro-Oncology Group, Institute of Oncology, Clínicalas Américas, Medellín, Colombia

References

[1] CBTRUS 2000-2004 data. United States population estimates by 5-year age group were obtained from United States census; estimates available at www.census.gov.

[2] Ries LAG, Melbert D, Krapcho M, et al (eds). SEER Cancer Statistics Review, 1975–2004, National Cancer Institute. Bethesda, MD, http://seer.cancer.gov/csr/1975_2004/, based on November 2006 SEER data submission, posted to the SEER web site, 2008

[3] Ferlay J, Bray F, PisaniP,et al. GLOBOCAN 2002: Cancer Incidence, Mortality and PrevalenceWorldwide, Version 2.0. IARC CancerBase No. 5. Lyon, IARCPress, 2004. Limited version available from: URL: http://www_depdb.iarc.fr/globocan2002.htm

[4] Stupp R, Roila F; ESMO Guidelines Working Group. Malignant glioma: ESMO clinical recommendations for diagnosis, treatment and follow-up. Ann Oncol. 2008; 19 (Suppl 2): 83-5.

[5] Gilbert MR. Designing clinical trials for brain tumors: the next generation. CurrOncol Rep 2007; 9: 49-54.

[6] Buckner JC. Factors influencing survival in high grade gliomas. SeminOncol 2003; 30: 10-4.

[7] Stupp R, MasonWP, van den Bent MJ, et al. Radiotherapy plus concomitant and adjuvant temozolomide for glioblastoma. N Engl J Med 2005; 352: 987-96.

[8] Wong ET, Hess KR, Gleason MJ, et al. Outcomes and prognostic factors in recurrent glioma patients enrolled onto phase II clinical trials. J ClinOncol 1999; 17: 2572-8.

[9] Gilbertson RJ, Rich JN. Making a tumour's bed: glioblastoma stem cells and the vascular niche. Nat Rev Cancer 2007; 7: 733-6.

[10] Nam DH, Park K, Suh YL, et al. Expression of VEGF and brain specific angiogenesis inhibitor-1 in glioblastoma: prognostic significance. Oncol Rep 2004; 11: 863-9.

[11] Knizetova P, Darling JL, Bartek J. Vascular endothelial growth factor in astroglioma stem cell biology and response to therapy. J Cell Mol Med 2008; 12: 111-25.

[12] Reya T, Morrison SJ, Clarke MF, et al. Stem cells, cancer, and cancer stem cells. Nature 2001; 414: 105-11.

[13] Sell S. Stem cell origin of cancer and differentiation therapy. Crit Rev OncolHematol 2004; 51: 1-28.

[14] Bonnet D, Dick JE. Human acute myeloid leukemia is organized as a hierarchy that originates from a primitive hematopoietic cell. Nature Med 1997; 3: 730-7.

[15] Nottebohm F. Neuronal replacement in adulthood. Ann NY AcadSci 1985; 457:143-161.

[16] Lie DC, Song H, Colamarino SA, et al. Neurogenesis in the adult brain: new strategies for central nervous system diseases. Annu Rev PharmacolToxicol 2004; 44: 399-421.

[17] Ming GL, Song H. Adult neurogenesis in the mammalian central nervous system. Annu Rev Neurosci 2005; 28: 223-50.

[18] Doetsch F, Caille I, Lim DA, et al. Subventricular zone astrocytes are neural stem cells in the adult mammalian brain. Cell 1999; 97: 703-16.

[19] Morshead CM. Neural stem cells in the adult mammalian forebrain: a relatively quiescent subpopulation of subependymal cells. Neuron 1994; 13: 1071-82.

[20] Sanai N, Tramontin AD, Quiñones-Hinojosa A, et al. Unique astrocyte ribbon in adult human brain contains neural stem cells but lacks chain migration. Nature 2004; 427: 740-4.

[21] Doetsch F, Garcia-Verdugo JM, Alvarez-Buylla A. Cellular composition and three-dimensional organization of the subventricular germinal zone in the adult mammalian brain. J Neurosci 2007; 17: 5046-61.

[22] Guerrero H, Chaichana K, Quiñones A et al. Neurosphere Culture and Human Organotypic Model to Evaluate Brain Tumor Stem Cells. Can St Cell; 2009;568(6):73-83.

[23] Galli R, Binda E, Orfanelli U, et al. Isolation and characterization of tumorigenic, stem-like neural precursors from human glioblastoma. Cancer Res 2004; 64: 7011-21.

[24] Kania G, Corbeil D, Fuchs J. Somatic stem cell marker prominin-1/CD133 is expressed in embryonic stem cell derived progenitors. Stem Cells 2001; 23: 791-804.

[25] Singh SK, Hawkins C, Clarke ID. Identification of human brain tumour initiating cells. Nature 2004; 432: 396-401.

[26] Bao S, Wu Q, McLendon RE. Glioma stem cells promote radioresistance by preferential activation of the DNA damage response. Nature 2006; 444: 756-60.

[27] Rich JN. Cancer stem cells in radiation resistance. Cancer Res 2007; 67:8980-4.

[28] Liu G, Yuan X, Zeng Z. Analysis of gene expression and chemoresistance of CD133+ cancer stem cells in glioblastoma. Mol Cancer 2006; 5: 67-78.

[29] Jin F, Zhao L, Guo YJ et al. Influence of Etoposide on anti-apoptotic and multidrug resistance-associated protein genes in CD133 positive U251 glioblastoma stem-like cells. Brain Res. 2010;8(1336):103-11.

[30] Wang J, Sakariassen P, Tsinkalovsky O et al. CD133 negative glioma cells form tumors in nude rats and give rise to CD133 positive cells. Int J Can. 2008;122:761–8.

[31] Ogden A, Waziri A, Lochhead R. Identification of A2B5+CD133- tumor-initiating cells in adult human gliomas. Neurosurgery. 2008;62:505–15.

[32] Schimmer AD. Inhibitor of apoptosis proteins: translating basic knowledge into clinical practice. Cancer Res 2004; 64: 7183-90.

[33] Vescovi AL, Galli R, Reynolds BA. Brain tumour stem cells. Nat Rev Cancer 2006; 426: 425-36.

[34] Dell'Albani P. Stem cell markers in gliomas. Neurochem Res 2008; 33: 2407-15.

[35] Gu H, Wang S, Messam CA, et al. Distribution of nestinimmunoreactivity in the normal adult human forebrain. Brain Res 2002; 943: 174-80.

[36] Holmin S, Almquist P, Lendahl U. Adult nestin expressing subependymal cells differentiate to astrocytes in response to brain injury. Eur J NeuroSci 1997; 9: 65-75.

[37] Dahlstrand J, Collins VP, Lendahl U. Expression of the class VI intermediate filament nestin in human central nervous system tumors. Cancer Res 1992; 52: 5334-41.

[38] Zhenju J, Lenhard R. Telomeres and telomerase in cancer stem cell. Eur J Cancer 2006; 42: 1197-203.

[39] Bi C, Fang J, Chen F et al. Chemoresistance of CD133(+) tumor stem cells from human brain glioma. Zhong Nan Da. 2007;32(4):568-73.

[40] Reilly K, Loisel D, Bronson R et al. Nf1; Trp53 mutant mice develop glioblastoma with evidence of strain-specific effects. Nat Genet. 2000;26:109–13.

[41] Bachoo RM, Maher EA, Ligon KL, et al. Epidermal growth factor receptor and Ink4a/Arf: convergent mechanisms governing terminal differentiation and transformation along the neural stem cell to astrocyte axis. Cancer Cell 2002; 1:269-77.

[42] Erlandsson A, Enarsson M, Forsberg-Nilsson K. Immature neurons from CNS stem cells proliferate in response to platelet-derived growth factor. J Neurosci 2001; 21: 3483-91.

[43] Ligon KL, Huillard E, Mehta S, et al. Olig2-regulated lineage-restricted pathway controls replication competence in neural stem cells and malignant glioma. Neuron 2007; 53: 503-17.

[44] Yoon K. Mind bomb 1-expressing intermediate progenitors generate notch signaling to maintain radial glial cells. Neuron. 2008;58:519–31.

[45] Mizutani K, Yoon K, Dang L et al. Differential Notch signalling distinguishes neural stem cells from intermediate progenitors. Nature. 2007;449:351–5.

[46] Corbin J. Regulation of neural progenitor cell development in the nervous system. J Neurochem. 2008;106:2272–87.

[47] Yoon K, Gaiano N. Notch signaling in the mammalian central nervous system: insights from mouse mutants. Nat Neurosci. 2005;8:709–15.

[48] Hoeck J, Jandke A, Blake S et al. Fbw7 controls neural stem cell differentiation and progenitor apoptosis via Notch and c-Jun. Nat Neurosc. 2010;13:1365–72.

[49] Hitoshi S, Seaberg RM, Koscik C, et al. Primitive neural stem cells from the mammalian epiblastdifferentiate to definitive neural stem cells under the control of Notch signalling. Genes Dev 2004; 18: 1806-11.

[50] Ferrari G, Bonini S, Uberti D et al. Targeting Notch pathway induces growth inhibition and differentiation of neuroblastoma cells. NeuroOncol. 2010;12(12):1231-43.

[51] Tanigaki K, Nogaki F, Takahashi J. Notch1 and Notch3 instructively restrict bFGF-responsive multipotent neural progenitor cells to an astroglial fate. Neuron 2001; 29: 45-55.

[52] Zhang XP, Zheng G, Zou L. Notch activation promotes cell proliferation and the formation of neural stem-like colonies in human glioma cells. Mol Cell Bioch 2008; 307:101-8.

[53] Purow BW, Haque RM, Noel MW, et al. Expression of Notch-1 and its ligands, Delta-like-1 and Jagged-1, is critical for glioma cell survival and proliferation. Cancer Res 2005; 65: 2353-63.

[54] Miele L. Notch Signaling. Clin Can Res 2006; 12: 1074-79.

[55] Singh SK, Clarke ID, Terasaki M, et al. Identification of a cancer stem cell in human brain tumors. Cancer Res 2003; 63: 5821-8.

[56] Assanah M. Lochhead R, Ogden A, et al. Glial progenitors in adult white matter are driven to form malignant gliomas by platelet-derived growth factor-expressing retroviruses. J Neurosci 2006; 26: 6781-90.

[57] Ayuso A, Moliterno JA, Kratovac S et al. Activated EGFR signaling increases proliferation, survival, and migration and blocks neuronal differentiation in post-natal neural stem cells. J Neurooncol. 2010;97(3):323-37.

[58] Garcion E, Halilagic A, Faissner A, et al. Generation of an environmental niche for neural stem cell development by the extracellular matrix molecule tenascin C. Development 2004; 131: 3423-32.

[59] Scadden DT. The stem-cell niche as an entity of action. Nature 2006; 441: 1075-79.

[60] Visvader JE, Lindeman GJ. Cancer stem cells in solid tumours: accumulating evidence and unresolved questions. Nat Rev Can 2008; 8: 755-68.

[61] Calabrese C, Poppleton H, Kocak M, et al. A perivascular niche for brain tumor stem cells. Cancer Cell 2007; 11: 69-82.

[62] Leon SP, Folkerth RD, Black PM. Microvessel density is a prognostic indicator for patients with astroglial brain tumors. Cancer 1996; 77: 362-72.

[63] Wang R, Chadalavada K, Wilshire J et al. Glioblastoma stem-like cells give rise to tumour endothelium. Nature. 2010;468:829–33.

[64] Bao S, Wu Q, Sathornsumetee S, et al. Stem cell-like glioma cells promote tumor angiogenesis through vascular endothelial growth factor. Cancer Res 2006; 66: 7843-48.

[65] Vredenburgh J, Desjardins A, Herndon JE 2nd et al. Bevacizumab plus irinotecan in recurrent glioblastomamultiforme. J ClinOncol. 2007;25(30):4722-9.

[66] Batchelor TT, Sorensen AG, di Tomaso E, et al. AZD2171, a pan-VEGF receptor tyrosine kinase inhibitor, normalizes tumor vasculature and alleviates edema in glioblastoma patients. Cancer Cell 2007; 11: 83-95.

[67] Batchelor T, Duda D, di Tomaso E et al. Phase II Study of Cediranib, an Oral Pan–Vascular Endothelial Growth Factor Receptor Tyrosine Kinase Inhibitor, in Patients With Recurrent Glioblastoma. J ClinOncol. 2007;25(30):4722-9.

[68] Loges S, Butzal M, Otten J, et al. Cilengitide inhibits proliferation and differentiation of human endothelial progenitor cells in vitro. BiochemBiophys Res Commun 2007; 357: 1016-20.

[69] Stupp R, Hegi ME, Neyns B et al. Phase I/IIa study of cilengitide and temozolomide with concomitant radiotherapy followed by cilengitide and temozolomide maintenance therapy in patients with newly diagnosed glioblastoma. J ClinOncol. 2010;28:2712-8.

[70] Tabatabai G, Weller M, Nabors B et al. Targeting integrins in malignant glioma. Target Oncol. 2010;5(3):175-81.

[71] Shaifer CA, Huang J, Lin PC. Glioblastoma cells incorporate into tumor vasculature and contribute to vascular radioresistance. Int J Cancer. 2010;127(9):2063-75.

[72] Sotelo C. Cellular and genetic regulation of the development of the cerebellar system. ProgNeurobiol 2004; 72: 295-339.

[73] Fan X, Eberhart CG. Medulloblastoma Stem Cells. J ClinOncol 2008; 26:2821-7.

[74] Wang VY, Rose MF, Zoghbi HY. Math1 expression redefines the rhombic lip derivatives and reveals novel lineages within the brainstem and cerebellum. Neuron 2005; 48: 31-43.

[75] Lee Y, Miller HL, Jensen P. A molecular fingerprint for medulloblastoma. Cancer Res 2003; 63: 5428-37.

[76] Dahmane N, Sanchez P, Gitton Y. The Sonic Hedgehog-Gli pathway regulates dorsal brain growth and tumorigenesis. Development 2001; 128: 5201-12.

[77] Yang Z, Ellis T, Markant S et al. Medulloblastoma Can Be Initiated by Deletion of Patched in Lineage-Restricted Progenitors or Stem Cells. Can Cell. 2008;14(2):135-45.

[78] Sasai K, Romer JT, Kimura H. Medulloblastomas derived from CXCR6 mutant mice respond to treatment with a smoothened inhibitor. Cancer Res 2007; 67: 3871-7.

[79] Schuller U, Rowitch DH. Beta-catenin function is required for cerebellar morphogenesis. Brain Res 2007; 1140: 161-9.

[80] Koch A, Hrychyk A, Hartmann W. Mutations of the Wnt antagonist AXIN2 (conductin) result in TCF-dependent transcription in medulloblastomas. Int J Cancer 2007; 121: 284-91.

[81] Clifford SC, Lusher ME, Lindsey JC. Wnt/Wingless pathway activation and chromosome 6 loss characterize a distinct molecular sub-group of medulloblastomas associated with a favorable prognosis. Cell Cycle 2006; 5: 2666-70.

[82] Dakubo GD, Mazerolle CJ, Wallace VA. Expression of Notch and Wnt pathway components and activation of Notch signaling in meduloblastomas from heterozygous patched mice. J Neurooncol 2006; 79: 221-7.

[83] Keith B, Simon MC. Hypoxia-inducible factors, stem cells, and cancer. Cell 2007; 129: 465-72.

[84] Read T, Fogarty M, Markant S et al. Identification of CD15 as a Marker for Tumor-Propagating Cells in a Mouse Model of Medulloblastoma. Can Cell. 2009:15:135–47.

[85] Beier D, Wischhusen J, Dietmaier W, et al. CD133 expression and cancer stem cells predict prognosis in high-grade oligodendroglial tumors. Brain Pathol 2008;18: 370-7.

[86] Zhang M, Song T, Yang L, et al. Nestin and CD133: valuable stem cell-specific markers for determining clinical outcome of glioma patients. J ExpClin Cancer Res 2008; 27: 85.

[87] Pallini R, Ricci L, Banna G et al.Cancer Stem Cell Analysis and Clinical Outcome in Patients with GlioblastomaMultiforme. ClinCancer Res 2008;14:8205-12.

[88] Spira AI, Carducci MA. Differentiation therapy. CurrOpinPharmacol 2003; 3: 338-43.

[89] Massard C, Deutsch E, Soria JC. Tumour stem cell-targeted treatment: elimination or differentiation. Ann Oncol 2006; 17: 1620-4.

[90] Nicolis SK. Cancer stem cells and "stemness" genes in neuro-oncology. Neurobiol Dis 2007; 25: 217-29.

[91] Clement V, Sanchez P, de Tribolet N, et al. HEDGEHOG–GLI1 signaling regulates human glioma growth, cancer stem cell self-renewal, and tumorigenicity. CurrBiol 2007; 17: 165-72.

[92] Chearwae W, Bright JJ. PPARgamma agonists inhibit growth and expansion of CD133+ brain tumour stem cells. Br J Cancer 2008; 99:2044-53.

[93] Beier D, Röhrl S, Pillai DR, et al. Temozolomide preferentially depletes cancer stem cells in glioblastoma. Cancer Res 2008; 68: 5706-15.

[94] Guzman ML. The sesquiterpene lactone parthenolide induces apoptosis of human acute myelogenous leukemia stem and progenitor cells. Blood 2005; 105: 4163-9.

[95] Piccirillo SG, Reynolds BA, Zanetti N, et al. Bone morphogenetic proteins inhibit the tumorigenic potential of human brain tumour-initiating cells. Nature 2006; 444: 761-5.

[96]   Dresemann G, Hosius C, Lilienthal J, et al. Treatment failure due to intracerebral stem cell-like behavior of glioblastoma (GB) cells: A reason for targeted maintenance therapy with imatinib (I) and hydroxyurea (H)? An analysis of study DE21 and DE40 (Ambrosia). J ClinOncol 2008; 26: 2048[Abstr].

[97]   Abouantoun TJ, Macdonald TJ. Imatinib blocks migration and invasion of medullo-blastoma cells by concurrently inhibiting activation of platelet-derived growth factor receptor and transactivation of epidermal growth factor receptor. Mol Cancer Ther. 2009;5:1-19.

[98]   Schatton T, Murphy GF, Frank NY, et al. Identification of cells initiating human melanomas. Nature 2008; 451: 345-9.

[99]   Hambardzumyan D, Becher OJ, Rosenblum MK, et al. PI3K pathway regulates survival of cancer stem cells residing in the perivascular niche following radiation in medulloblastoma in vivo. Genes Dev 2008; 22: 436-48.

[100] Lu J, Zhang F, Zhao D, et al. ATRA-inhibited proliferation in glioma cells is associated with subcellular redistribution of beta-catenin via up-regulation of Axin. J Neurooncol 2008; 87: 271-7.

[101] Spiller SE, Ditzler SH, Pullar BJ, et al. Response of preclinical medulloblastoma models to combination therapy with 13-cis retinoic acid and suberoylanilidehydroxamic acid (SAHA). J Neurooncol 2008; 87: 133-41.

[102] Elisabeth CM, Leigh J, Kesari S, et al. Efficacy of the HSP90 inhibitor 17-AAG in human glioma cell lines and tumorigenic glioma stem cells. NeuroOncol 2009; 11: 109-21.

[103] Bar EE, Chaudhry A, Lin A, et al. Cyclopamine-mediated hedgehog pathway inhibition depletes stem-like cancer cells in glioblastoma. Stem Cells 2007; 25: 2524-33.

[104] Lee J, Son MJ, Woolard K, et al. Epigenetic-mediated dysfunction of the bone morphogenetic protein pathway inhibits differentiation of glioblastoma-initiating cells. Cancer Cell 2008; 13: 69-80.

[105] Di Tomaso T, Mazzoleni S, Wang E, et al. Immunobiological characterization of cancer stem cells isolated from glioblastoma patients. Clin Cancer Res 2010; 16: 800-13.

[106] Xu Q, Liu G, Yuan X, et al. Antigen-specific T-cell response from dendritic cell vaccination using cancer stem-like cell-associated antigens. Stem Cells 2009; 27: 1734-40.

[107] Castellino R, Muh C, Durden D. PI-3 Kinase-PTEN Signaling Node: An Intercept Point for the Control of Angiogenesis. Curr Pharm Des. 2009;15(4):380-8.

[108] Kast R, Belda C. Suppressing Glioblastoma Stem Cell Function by Aldehyde Dehydrogenase Inhibition with Chloramphenicol or Disulfiram as a New Treatment Adjunct. Curr St Cell Res Ther. 2009;4:314-7.

Chapter 9

Nestin: Neural Stem/Progenitor Cell Marker in Brain Tumors

Yoko Matsuda, Hisashi Yoshimura,
Taeko Suzuki and Toshiyuki Ishiwata

Additional information is available at the end of the chapter

1. Introduction

Glioblastomas are the most common primary malignant neoplasms in the adult brain, and have the characteristics of glial cells [1]. The WHO histopathological classification guidelines categorize gliomas according to their histopathological grades; low-grade gliomas are not anaplastic and are associated with a favorable patient prognosis, while high-grade gliomas exhibit increased cellularity, nuclear atypia, mitotic activity, microvascular proliferation, and necrosis. Glioblastomas are the highest grade of the gliomas. Surgical treatment is the main therapy used for glioblastomas, with radiotherapy and chemotherapy performed as adjuvant care. Despite intensive research and recent advances in treatment, the prognosis for patients with glioblastoma remains poor, with a five-year survival rate of approximately 3% [2, 3]. In addition to having rapid growth rates, glioblastomas aggressively invade the adjacent normal brain tissues, they are often surgically unresectable, and recurrent glioblastomas are resistant to conventional radiotherapy and chemotherapy.

Nestin is a class VI intermediate filament protein that was first described as a neural stem/progenitor cell marker [4, 5]. Neuroepithelial stem cells can differentiate into neurons, oligodendrocytes, and astrocytes, and nestin has been shown to be down-regulated or to completely disappear during such differentiation. Nestin-positive neuroepithelial stem cells are detected in the subventricular zone of the human adult brain and they remain mitotically active throughout adulthood [6]. Unlike other intermediate filament proteins, nestin plays important roles in cellular processes, including stemness, migration, and cell cycle regulation.

Nestin expression has been reported in various types of tumor cells originating from the central nervous system, including glioblastomas. Several reports have indicated a close relationship between neuroepithelial stem cells and glioblastoma cells at their origin because both cell types express the same stem cell markers, such as CD133 and nestin. High-grade gliomas express higher nestin levels compared to low-grade gliomas [7, 8]. We have reported that knockdown of nestin using short hairpin RNA (shRNA) suppressed cell growth, migration, and invasion [9]; therefore, nestin may serve as a novel candidate for molecular targeted therapy for glioblastomas. In the present chapter, we summarize the available data regarding the expression and roles of nestin in normal brain tissues and brain tumor tissues, and discuss the possibility of using nestin as a novel therapeutic target in brain tumors, mainly for glioblastomas.

2. Structure and characterization of nestin

Nestin is a large protein (>1600 amino acids) that contains a short N-terminal and an unusually long C-terminal. It interacts with other intermediate filament proteins, including vimentin, desmin, and internexin, to form heterodimers and mixed polymers; however, in contrast to other intermediate filament proteins, nestin cannot form homopolymers [10]. The nestin gene has four exons and three introns; in humans, neural cell-specific expression is reportedly regulated by the second intron, whereas nestin expression in tumor endothelium is enhanced by the first intron [11]. Nestin is known to be phosphorylated on Thr316 by cdc2 kinase [12] and/or cyclin-dependent kinase 5 [13], and to modulate mitosis-associated cytoplasmic reorganization during mitosis. However, the roles of glycosylation of nestin have not been closely examined [14].

During early stages of development, nestin is expressed in dividing cells in the central nervous system (CNS), peripheral nervous system, and in myogenic and other tissues. During differentiation in normal brain tissue, nestin expression is downregulated and replaced by expression of tissue-specific intermediate filament proteins; therefore, nesting is widely used as a neuronal stem cell marker. Nestin is also expressed in immature non-neuronal cells and progenitor cells in normal tissues [15-17]. High levels of nestin expression have been detected in oligodendroglial lineage cells, ependymocytes, Sertoli cells, enteroglia, hair follicle cells, podocytes of renal glomeruli, pancreatic stellate cells, pericytes, islets, optic nerve, and odontoblasts [18-23].

In pathological conditions, nestin is re-expressed during repair processes, as well as in various neoplasms and proliferating endothelial cells. Nestin expression has been observed in repair processes in the CNS, muscle, liver, and infarcted myocardium [24-26]. Furthermore, increased nestin expression has been reported in various tumor cells, including CNS tumors, pancreatic cancer, gastrointestinal stromal tumors (GISTs), prostate cancers, breast cancers, malignant melanomas, dermatofibrosarcoma protuberances, and thyroid tumors [27-31]. In several tumors, expression of nestin has been reported to be closely correlated with poor prognosis. Nestin is specifically expressed in proliferating small-sized vascular endothelial cells in glioblastomas and in colorectal, prostate, and pancreatic cancers [7, 32-34].

3. Nestin in normal fetal and adult brain tissues

Many lines of evidence have shown nestin-positive brain cells to be neural stem/progenitor cells; therefore, a great deal of research has involved the use of nestin to detect neural stem cells [35-37]. Children, but not adult humans, exhibit nestin-positive cells in the subventricular zone of the third ventricle [6], and the human embryonic midbrain stem cell line NGC-407 showed degradation of nestin after induction of differentiation [38]. However, in adult mice, nestin-positive cells were detected in CA2 lesions of the hippocampus after transient ischemia [39]. Another study reported that nestin-positive neuroepithelial stem cells are detected in the subventricular zone of the human adult brain and remain mitotically active throughout adulthood [40]. Nestin has been used for research in the field of neural progenitor cells; for example, neural progenitor cell-specific gene transfection was successfully performed using a nestin-driven gene transfection system [41-46]. A recent study has shown that nestin is also a stem/progenitor cell marker in the pituitary gland [47].

4. Nestin in various types of brain tumors

Nestin expression in brain tumor cells has been reported in schwannomas [48], ependymomas [49, 50], neurocytomas [51], adamantinomatous craniopharyngiomas [52], pituitary adenomas [53], medulloblastomas [54-59], oligodendrogliomas [60], and glioblastomas [7, 8, 48, 61] (Table 1). Tissue microarrays of 257 brain tumors have revealed frequent nestin expression in gliomas and schwannomas [48]. Another analysis included 379 tumors, and the results further revealed that nestin immunoreactivity is associated with poor outcome in intracranial ependymomas, and that nestin is an independent marker for poor progression-free survival and overall survival [49].

Expression of nestin has also been reported in tanycytic ependymoma, a rare variant of ependymoma [50], and central neurocytoma cases express nestin, as determined by PCR [51]. Co-expression of nestin, microtubule-associated protein 2 (MAP2), and GFAP has been reported in adamantinomatous craniopharyngiomas [52]. In pituitary adenomas, CD133-positive cells ubiquitously co-express CD34, nestin, and VEGFR2, and may play a role in the neovascularization of tumors [53]. Human medulloblastoma cell lines [54] and medulloblastoma stem cells [55-58] express nestin, and secreted protein acidic and rich in cysteine (SPARC) has been shown to induce neuronal differentiation in medulloblastoma cells with elevations of nestin, NeuN, and neurofilament [59]. One study found that oligodendrogliomas express no or weak nestin, but high Olig2 and alpha-internexin [60]. Oligoastrocytomas moderately express nestin, while astrocytoma and glioblastoma strongly express nestin. Nestin is an intermediate filament protein and is localized in the cytoplasm in most brain tumors; however, in human neuroblastoma and medulloblastoma cell lines, nestin has been observed in nuclei [62], suggesting that nestin may directly bind to DNA or intranucleic proteins. Altogether, these findings demonstrate that nestin is expressed in a wide variety of brain tumors and that this expression correlates with their functions or cell behaviors.

Brain tumors	Expression pattern and roles
Schwannomas	Frequent nestin expression [48]
Ependymomas	Poor progression-free survival and overall survival [49]
Neurocytomas [51]	N/D
Adamantinomatous craniopharyngiomas	Expressed in the invasion niche [52]
Pituitary adenomas	Coexpressed with CD133 [53]
Medulloblastomas	Expressed in tumor stem cells [55-58]
Oligodendrogliomas [60]	N/D
Gliomas	High grade [7,8]
	Worse overall survival [48,61]
Glioblastomas	Infiltration into surrounding tissue [8]
	Tumor stem cells [72-77]
N/D: Not determined.	

Table 1. Expression and roles of nestin in brain tumors

5. Nestin in glioblastoma

5.1. Nestin in low-grade gliomas and glioblastomas

Immunohistochemical analysis has demonstrated nestin expression in the cytoplasm of glioblastoma cells (Figure 1). Large-scale and multicenter studies have shown high immunoreactivity of nestin in glioma cases to be correlated with high grade [7, 8] and worse overall survival [48, 61] (Table 1). Furthermore, expression of nestin and MIB-1 labeling indices in immunohistochemical analyses may correlate with aggressiveness of pilocytic astrocytoma and pilomyxoid astrocytoma [63]. An analysis of several stem cell markers—including CD133, nestin, B lymphoma Mo-MLV insertion region 1 homolog (BMI-1), Maternal embryonic leucine zipper kinase (MELK), and Notch 1-4—was performed using quantitative RT-PCR in 42 glioblastoma samples; MELK was most upregulated, followed by nestin [64]. In contrast, others have reported that nestin immunoreactivity is mostly due to an acute glial reaction and is not specific to the neoplasm [65], and that nestin expression in gliomas does not correlate with prognosis [66].

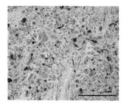

Figure 1. Expression of nestin in glioblastomas. Bar, 100 μm

Immunostaining of nestin in glioblastoma cells has been demonstrated to delineate between invading tumor and the adjacent gray and white matter; therefore, nestin is considered to be a useful marker for examining the infiltration of glioblastomas into surrounding tissues [8]. Furthermore, knockdown of nestin in human glioblastoma cells has been shown to suppress cell migration and invasion, and to increase F-actin expression and cell adhesion to extracellular matrices [9].

Nestin-positive non-tumorous brain cells migrate into the glioblastoma cells and delay astrocytic or elongated bipolar morphology and glomerulus-like microvasculature [67]; therefore, nestin-positive cells have been considered an important component of the tumor microenvironment. CD133-positive and nestin-positive niches are perivascularly localized in all glioma tissues, and the presence of these niches increases significantly with increasing tumor grade [68]. Mice were engineered to co-express platelet-derived growth factor B receptor and Bcl-2 under the control of the glioneuronal-specific nestin promoter, and this resulted in the development of low- and high-grade gliomas [69]. Another study found that human glioblastoma subclones characterized by high nestin levels formed tumors in vivo at a significantly faster rate than subclones with low nestin expression, suggesting that induction of nestin plays an important role in glioblastoma carcinogenesis [70]. However, the opposite result has also been reported [71].

5.2. Nestin in glioma stem cells

Cancer stem cells appear to be responsible for tumor metastasis, resistance to radiotherapy and chemotherapy, and disease relapse; thus, their analysis and therapeutic targeting are believed to be crucial. Many studies have shown that there is a small population of cancer stem cells in glioblastomas, and that nestin is one of the stem/progenitor cell markers of glioblastomas [72-77]. CD133, Oct4, Sox2, and Nanog have also been considered to be stem cell markers in glioblastomas [78, 79]. However, CD133-negative and nestin-negative glioblastoma cells show tumorigenic potential in vivo [71]; thus, there remains some controversy over which specific markers should be used to detect glioblastoma stem cells. An in vitro study has shown that neurospheres of glioblastoma cells exhibit high expressions of nestin, CD133, and Oct4 compared to the expressions in monolayer cells [80]. One study reported that radiation induces increased expressions of stem cell markers, including nestin, CD133, and Musashi [81]; in contrast, another study has shown that radiation induced accumulation of CD133-positive glioblastoma cells, but not nestin [82]. Glioblastoma stem cells are maintained in vivo in a niche characterized by hypoxia, and hypoxia reportedly increases the expressions of nestin, CD133, podoplanin, and Bmi-1 [83]. Together, these available data suggest that there is close relationship between nestin and stemness in glioblastoma.

Expression of nestin in cancer stem cells of glioblastoma may indicate the origin and function of these cells. Potential cancer stem cell origins include migration of neural stem cells toward the tumor, migration of mesenchymal stem cells from bone marrow, or dedifferentiation of tumor cells [84]; each of these hypotheses have been proven experimentally. In brain tumors, long-term cultured human neural stem cells undergo spontaneous transformation to tumor-initiating cells [37]. In contrast, Nanog promotes dedifferentiation of p53-deficient mouse astrocytes into glioblastoma stem cells [85]. These results indicate that glioblastoma stem cells may arise from both the transformation of nestin-positive neural stem cells and differentiated astrocytes. Retinoic acid treatment for glioblastoma stem cells was demonstrated to reduce the expression of neural stem cell markers, such as nestin, CD133, Msi-1, and Sox-2 [86].

Xenografts developed from human anaplastic astrocytoma and glioblastoma tumor-derived spheres in the brain of a nude mouse revealed co-expression of PCNA, VCAM-1, caspase-3, and nestin [87]. Cells positive for both caspase-3 and nestin were located adjacent to or around the blood vessels. Glioblastoma stem cells expressed nestin/CD31 or CD133/CD31, and these cells were capable of differentiating into endothelial cells [88]. Dong et al. have shown that human glioma stem/progenitor cells transdifferentiate into vascular endothelial cells in vitro and in vivo [89]. Glioblastoma stem cells have close relationships with the angiogenic switch, intratumor hypoxia, and the neoplastic microvascular network. These findings provide new insights for targeted therapy against glioblastomas.

5.3. Regulation of nestin in glioblastoma cells

Glioblastomas usually show hyperactivation of the PI3K-Akt pathway. Exogeneous expression of the Akt-binding domain of Girdin inhibits its Akt-mediated phosphorylation, and reportedly diminishes migration and the expression of the stem cell markers nestin and SOX2 [90]. Nestin expression in glioblastomas is correlated with proangiogenic chemokines (CXCL12 and its receptor CXCR4) and growth factors (VEGF and PDGF-B and its receptor PDGFRbeta) [91]. Hypoxia and radiation are both inducers of stem cells, and were associated with increased expression of nestin [81, 83]. In glioblastoma cases, a 9-gene profile that included podoplanin and insulin-like growth factor binding protein 2 was found to predict the prognosis, and was also positively associated with expressions of nestin and CD133 [92]. Additionally, the enhancer lesion of nestin is known to be located in the second intron in neural cells, and this lesion is highly conserved in mouse, rat, and human [93].

5.4. Nestin in interstitial tissues and angiogenesis of glioblastoma

Glioblastoma-conditioned medium has been shown to induce human mesenchymal stem cells (hMSCs) to increase expressions of nestin, CD151, VE-cadherin, desmin, α-smooth muscle actin, and nerval/glial antigen 2—indicating pericyte-like differentiation, rather than differentiation to endothelial cells or smooth muscle cells [94]. hMSCs migrate towards glioblastoma and are incorporated into tumor microvessels.

Much evidence has shown that expression of nestin in vascular endothelial cells is associated with proliferation and angiogenesis [32, 95-98]. In glioblastomas, expression of nestin in both tumor cells and endothelial cells was increased according to increasing tumor grade [7]. A recent study has indicated that the capillaries in gliomas may come from the differentiation of glioblastoma stem cells, and that the glioblastoma stem cells are accumulated around the capillaries [99]. In contrast, CD105 has been proposed to be a more useful marker of tumor angiogenesis in glioblastomas than nestin [100]. The morphology of nestin-positive cells in brain tumors is reportedly more typical of neural stem cells, and less than 0.1% of these cells co-express the endothelial marker CD34 [101].

5.5. Nestin as a therapeutic target for glioblastoma

We have reported that knockdown of nestin using shRNA suppresses cell migration and invasion [9]. Lu et al. demonstrated that blocking the expression of nestin in glioblastomas via intratumor injection of shRNA significantly slowed tumor growth and volume [70]; therefore, nestin may serve as a novel candidate for molecular targeted therapy for glioblastomas [9]. The phytoalexin resveratrol suppresses cell growth, migration, invasion, and expression of nestin in glioblastoma cells [102]. It has been shown that peptides can bind to a nestin isotype that is specifically expressed in glioma stem cells, which enables them to target nestin-positive cells in human glioma tissue [103]. Future studies should focus on developing delivery systems to target these anti-nestin reagents to brain tumors, and on the estimation of the side-effects for normal brain stem cells that express nestin.

6. Conclusion

The neuronal stem cell marker nestin regulates cell growth, migration, invasion, and stemness, and has been found to be expressed in a wide variety of brain tumors. Nestin may be a candidate for the development of promising therapeutic and diagnostic modalities for glioblastoma.

Acknowledgements

The authors thank Dr. Zenya Naito, Mr. Yuji Yanagisawa, Ms. Yoko Kawamoto, Ms. Kiyoko Kawahara, and Ms. Megumi Murase (Departments of Pathology and Integrative Oncological Pathology) for helpful discussions, and Ms. Yuko Ono (Departments of Pathology and Integrative Oncological Pathology) for preparing the manuscript.

Author details

Yoko Matsuda, Hisashi Yoshimura, Taeko Suzuki and Toshiyuki Ishiwata*

*Address all correspondence to: ishiwata@nms.ac.jp

Departments of Pathology and Integrative Oncological Pathology, Nippon Medical School, Bunkyo-ku, Toky, Japan

References

[1] Louis DN, Ohgaki H, Wiestler OD, Cavenee WK, Burger PC, Jouvet A, Scheithauer BW, Kleihues P. The 2007 WHO classification of tumours of the central nervous system. Acta Neuropathol 2007;114(2):97-109.

[2] Bondy ML, Scheurer ME, Malmer B, Barnholtz-Sloan JS, Davis FG, Il'yasova D, Kruchko C, McCarthy BJ, Rajaraman P, Schwartzbaum JA, Sadetzki S, Schlehofer B, Tihan T, Wiemels JL, Wrensch M, Buffler PA. Brain tumor epidemiology: consensus from the Brain Tumor Epidemiology Consortium. Cancer 2008;113(7 Suppl):1953-68.

[3] Brem SS, Bierman PJ, Black P, Blumenthal DT, Brem H, Chamberlain MC, Chiocca EA, DeAngelis LM, Fenstermaker RA, Fine HA, Friedman A, Glass J, Grossman SA, Heimberger AB, Junck L, Levin V, Loeffler JJ, Maor MH, Narayana A, Newton HB, Olivi A, Portnow J, Prados M, Raizer JJ, Rosenfeld SS, Shrieve DC, Sills AK, Jr., Spence AM, Vrionis FD. Central nervous system cancers: Clinical Practice Guidelines in Oncology. J Natl Compr Canc Netw 2005;3(5):644-90.

[4] Lendahl U, Zimmerman LB, McKay RD. CNS stem cells express a new class of intermediate filament protein. Cell 1990;60(4):585-95.

[5] Ishiwata T, Matsuda Y, Naito Z. Nestin in gastrointestinal and other cancers: effects on cells and tumor angiogenesis. World J Gastroenterol 2011;17(4):409-18.

[6] Dahiya S, Lee da Y, Gutmann DH. Comparative characterization of the human and mouse third ventricle germinal zones. J Neuropathol Exp Neurol 2011;70(7):622-33.

[7] Hlobilkova A, Ehrmann J, Knizetova P, Krejci V, Kalita O, Kolar Z. Analysis of VEGF, Flt-1, Flk-1, nestin and MMP-9 in relation to astrocytoma pathogenesis and progression. Neoplasma 2009;56(4):284-90.

[8] Kitai R, Horita R, Sato K, Yoshida K, Arishima H, Higashino Y, Hashimoto N, Takeuchi H, Kubota T, Kikuta K. Nestin expression in astrocytic tumors delineates tumor infiltration. Brain Tumor Pathol 2010;27(1):17-21.

[9] Ishiwata T, Teduka K, Yamamoto T, Kawahara K, Matsuda Y, Naito Z. Neuroepithelial stem cell marker nestin regulates the migration, invasion and growth of human gliomas. Oncol Rep 2011;26(1):91-9.

[10] Steinert PM, Chou YH, Prahlad V, Parry DA, Marekov LN, Wu KC, Jang SI, Gold-man RD. A high molecular weight intermediate filament-associated protein in BHK-21 cells is nestin, a type VI intermediate filament protein. Limited co-assembly in vitro to form heteropolymers with type III vimentin and type IV alpha-internexin. J Biol Chem 1999;274(14):9881-90.

[11] Aihara M, Sugawara K, Torii S, Hosaka M, Kurihara H, Saito N, Takeuchi T. Angiogenic endothelium-specific nestin expression is enhanced by the first intron of the nestin gene. Lab Invest 2004;84(12):1581-92.

[12] Sahlgren CM, Mikhailov A, Hellman J, Chou YH, Lendahl U, Goldman RD, Eriksson JE. Mitotic reorganization of the intermediate filament protein nestin involves phosphorylation by cdc2 kinase. J Biol Chem 2001;276(19):16456-63.

[13] Sahlgren CM, Mikhailov A, Vaittinen S, Pallari HM, Kalimo H, Pant HC, Eriksson JE. Cdk5 regulates the organization of Nestin and its association with p35. Mol Cell Biol 2003;23(14):5090-106.

[14] Grigelioniene G, Blennow M, Torok C, Fried G, Dahlin I, Lendahl U, Lagercrantz H. Cerebrospinal fluid of newborn infants contains a deglycosylated form of the intermediate filament nestin. Pediatr Res 1996;40(6):809-14.

[15] Sejersen T, Lendahl U. Transient expression of the intermediate filament nestin during skeletal muscle development. J Cell Sci 1993;106 (Pt 4):1291-300.

[16] Frojdman K, Pelliniemi LJ, Lendahl U, Virtanen I, Eriksson JE. The intermediate filament protein nestin occurs transiently in differentiating testis of rat and mouse. Differentiation 1997;61(4):243-9.

[17] Terling C, Rass A, Mitsiadis TA, Fried K, Lendahl U, Wroblewski J. Expression of the intermediate filament nestin during rodent tooth development. Int J Dev Biol 1995;39(6):947-56.

[18] Yang J, Bian W, Gao X, Chen L, Jing N. Nestin expression during mouse eye and lens development. Mech Dev 2000;94(1-2):287-91.

[19] Almazan G, Vela JM, Molina-Holgado E, Guaza C. Re-evaluation of nestin as a marker of oligodendrocyte lineage cells. Microsc Res Tech 2001;52(6):753-65.

[20] Amoh Y, Li L, Yang M, Moossa AR, Katsuoka K, Penman S, Hoffman RM. Nascent blood vessels in the skin arise from nestin-expressing hair-follicle cells. Proc Natl Acad Sci U S A 2004;101(36):13291-5.

[21] Lardon J, Rooman I, Bouwens L. Nestin expression in pancreatic stellate cells and angiogenic endothelial cells. Histochem Cell Biol 2002;117(6):535-40.

[22] Takano T, Rutka JT, Becker LE. Overexpression of nestin and vimentin in ependymal cells in hydrocephalus. Acta Neuropathol 1996;92(1):90-7.

[23] Ishizaki M, Ishiwata T, Adachi A, Tamura N, Ghazizadeh M, Kitamura H, Sugisaki Y, Yamanaka N, Naito Z, Fukuda Y. Expression of nestin in rat and human glomerular podocytes. J Submicrosc Cytol Pathol 2006;38(2-3):193-200.

[24] Niki T, Pekny M, Hellemans K, Bleser PD, Berg KV, Vaeyens F, Quartier E, Schuit F, Geerts A. Class VI intermediate filament protein nestin is induced during activation of rat hepatic stellate cells. Hepatology 1999;29(2):520-7.

[25] Lin RC, Matesic DF, Marvin M, McKay RD, Brustle O. Re-expression of the intermediate filament nestin in reactive astrocytes. Neurobiol Dis 1995;2(2):79-85.

[26] El-Helou V, Dupuis J, Proulx C, Drapeau J, Clement R, Gosselin H, Villeneuve L, Manganas L, Calderone A. Resident nestin+ neural-like cells and fibers are detected in normal and damaged rat myocardium. Hypertension 2005;46(5):1219-25.

[27] Yamada H, Takano T, Ito Y, Matsuzuka F, Miya A, Kobayashi K, Yoshida H, Watanabe M, Iwatani Y, Miyauchi A. Expression of nestin mRNA is a differentiation marker in thyroid tumors. Cancer Lett 2009;280(1):61-4.

[28] Strojnik T, Rosland GV, Sakariassen PO, Kavalar R, Lah T. Neural stem cell markers, nestin and musashi proteins, in the progression of human glioma: correlation of nestin with prognosis of patient survival. Surg Neurol 2007;68(2):133-43; discussion 43-4.

[29] Brychtova S, Fiuraskova M, Hlobilkova A, Brychta T, Hirnak J. Nestin expression in cutaneous melanomas and melanocytic nevi. J Cutan Pathol 2007;34(5):370-5.

[30] Tsujimura T, Makiishi-Shimobayashi C, Lundkvist J, Lendahl U, Nakasho K, Sugihara A, Iwasaki T, Mano M, Yamada N, Yamashita K, Toyosaka A, Terada N. Expression of the intermediate filament nestin in gastrointestinal stromal tumors and interstitial cells of Cajal. Am J Pathol 2001;158(3):817-23.

[31] Li H, Cherukuri P, Li N, Cowling V, Spinella M, Cole M, Godwin AK, Wells W, DiRenzo J. Nestin is expressed in the basal/myoepithelial layer of the mammary gland and is a selective marker of basal epithelial breast tumors. Cancer Res 2007;67(2): 501-10.

[32] Gravdal K, Halvorsen OJ, Haukaas SA, Akslen LA. Proliferation of immature tumor vessels is a novel marker of clinical progression in prostate cancer. Cancer Res 2009;69(11):4708-15.

[33] Teranishi N, Naito Z, Ishiwata T, Tanaka N, Furukawa K, Seya T, Shinji S, Tajiri T. Identification of neovasculature using nestin in colorectal cancer. Int J Oncol 2007;30(3):593-603.

[34] Yamahatsu K, Matsuda Y, Ishiwata T, Uchida E, Naito Z. Nestin as a novel therapeutic target for pancreatic cancer via tumor angiogenesis. Int J Oncol 2012;40(5):1345-57.

[35] Liu L, Shi M, Wang L, Hou S, Wu Z, Zhao G, Deng Y. Ndrg2 expression in neurogenic germinal zones of embryonic and postnatal mouse brain. J Mol Histol 2012; 43 (1): 27-35.

[36] Romero-Grimaldi C, Murillo-Carretero M, Lopez-Toledano MA, Carrasco M, Castro C, Estrada C. ADAM-17/tumor necrosis factor-alpha-converting enzyme inhibits neurogenesis and promotes gliogenesis from neural stem cells. Stem Cells 2011;29(10):1628-39.

[37] Wu W, He Q, Li X, Zhang X, Lu A, Ge R, Zhen H, Chang AE, Li Q, Shen L. Long-term cultured human neural stem cells undergo spontaneous transformation to tumor-initiating cells. Int J Biol Sci 2011;7(6):892-901.

[38] Khan Z, Akhtar M, Ekstrom TJ. HDAC inhibitor 4-phenylbutyrate preserves immature phenotype of human embryonic midbrain stem cells: implications for the involvement of DNA methyltransferase. Int J Mol Med 2011;28(6):977-83.

[39] Wang H, Imamura Y, Ishibashi R, Chandana EP, Yamamoto M, Noda M. The Reck tumor suppressor protein alleviates tissue damage and promotes functional recovery after transient cerebral ischemia in mice. J Neurochem 2010;115(2):385-98.

[40] Kaneko Y, Sakakibara S, Imai T, Suzuki A, Nakamura Y, Sawamoto K, Ogawa Y, Toyama Y, Miyata T, Okano H. Musashi1: an evolutionarily conserved marker for CNS progenitor cells including neural stem cells. Dev Neurosci 2000;22(1-2):139-53.

[41] Seok SH, Na YR, Han JH, Kim TH, Jung H, Lee BH, Emelyanov A, Parinov S, Park JH. Cre/loxP-regulated transgenic zebrafish model for neural progenitor-specific oncogenic Kras expression. Cancer Sci 2010;101(1):149-54.

[42] Goto J, Talos DM, Klein P, Qin W, Chekaluk YI, Anderl S, Malinowska IA, Di Nardo A, Bronson RT, Chan JA, Vinters HV, Kernie SG, Jensen FE, Sahin M, Kwiatkowski DJ. Regulable neural progenitor-specific Tsc1 loss yields giant cells with organellar dysfunction in a model of tuberous sclerosis complex. Proc Natl Acad Sci U S A 2011;108(45):E1070-9.

[43] Nagy JI, Lynn BD, Tress O, Willecke K, Rash JE. Connexin26 expression in brain parenchymal cells demonstrated by targeted connexin ablation in transgenic mice. Eur J Neurosci 2011;34(2):263-71.

[44] Wey A, Knoepfler PS. c-myc and N-myc promote active stem cell metabolism and cycling as architects of the developing brain. Oncotarget 2010;1(2):120-30.

[45] Tanori M, Santone M, Mancuso M, Pasquali E, Leonardi S, Di Majo V, Rebessi S, Saran A, Pazzaglia S. Developmental and oncogenic effects of insulin-like growth factor-I in Ptc1+/- mouse cerebellum. Mol Cancer 2010;9:53.

[46] See WL, Miller JP, Squatrito M, Holland E, Resh MD, Koff A. Defective DNA double-strand break repair underlies enhanced tumorigenesis and chromosomal instability in p27-deficient mice with growth factor-induced oligodendrogliomas. Oncogene 2010;29(12):1720-31.

[47] Florio T. Adult pituitary stem cells: from pituitary plasticity to adenoma development. Neuroendocrinology 2011;94(4):265-77.

[48] Arai H, Ikota H, Sugawara KI, Nobusawa S, Hirato J, Nakazato Y. Nestin expression in brain tumors: its utility for pathological diagnosis and correlation with the prognosis of high-grade gliomas. Brain Tumor Pathol 2012; 29 (3): 160-7.

[49] Milde T, Hielscher T, Witt H, Kool M, Mack SC, Deubzer HE, Oehme I, Lodrini M, Benner A, Taylor MD, von Deimling A, Kulozik AE, Pfister SM, Witt O, Korshunov A. Nestin Expression Identifies Ependymoma Patients with Poor Outcome. Brain Pathol 2012.

[50] Zhang S, Wang X, Zhang Z, Chen Y. Tanycytic ependymoma arising from the right lateral ventricle: a case report and review of the literature. Neuropathology 2008;28(4):427-32.

[51] Paek SH, Shin HY, Kim JW, Park SH, Son JH, Kim DG. Primary culture of central neurocytoma: a case report. J Korean Med Sci 2010;25(5):798-803.

[52] Burghaus S, Holsken A, Buchfelder M, Fahlbusch R, Riederer BM, Hans V, Blumcke I, Buslei R. A tumor-specific cellular environment at the brain invasion border of adamantinomatous craniopharyngiomas. Virchows Arch 2010;456(3):287-300.

[53] Yunoue S, Arita K, Kawano H, Uchida H, Tokimura H, Hirano H. Identification of CD133+ cells in pituitary adenomas. Neuroendocrinology 2011;94(4):302-12.

[54] Kim YH, Cho SH, Lee SJ, Choi SA, Phi JH, Kim SK, Wang KC, Cho BK, Kim CY. Growth-inhibitory effect of neurotrophin-3-secreting adipose tissue-derived mesenchymal stem cells on the D283-MED human medulloblastoma cell line. J Neurooncol 2012;106(1):89-98.

[55] Huang X, Ketova T, Litingtung Y, Chiang C. Isolation, enrichment, and maintenance of medulloblastoma stem cells. J Vis Exp 2010(43).

[56] Pistollato F, Rampazzo E, Persano L, Abbadi S, Frasson C, Denaro L, D'Avella D, Panchision DM, Della Puppa A, Scienza R, Basso G. Interaction of hypoxia-inducible factor-1alpha and Notch signaling regulates medulloblastoma precursor proliferation and fate. Stem Cells 2010;28(11):1918-29.

[57] Yu CC, Chiou GY, Lee YY, Chang YL, Huang PI, Cheng YW, Tai LK, Ku HH, Chiou SH, Wong TT. Medulloblastoma-derived tumor stem-like cells acquired resistance to TRAIL-induced apoptosis and radiosensitivity. Childs Nerv Syst 2010;26(7):897-904.

[58] Sutter R, Shakhova O, Bhagat H, Behesti H, Sutter C, Penkar S, Santuccione A, Bernays R, Heppner FL, Schuller U, Grotzer M, Moch H, Schraml P, Marino S. Cerebellar stem cells act as medulloblastoma-initiating cells in a mouse model and a neural stem cell signature characterizes a subset of human medulloblastomas. Oncogene 2010;29(12):1845-56.

[59] Bhoopathi P, Chetty C, Dontula R, Gujrati M, Dinh DH, Rao JS, Lakka SS. SPARC stimulates neuronal differentiation of medulloblastoma cells via the Notch1/STAT3 pathway. Cancer Res 2011;71(14):4908-19.

[60] Durand K, Guillaudeau A, Pommepuy I, Mesturoux L, Chaunavel A, Gadeaud E, Porcheron M, Moreau JJ, Labrousse F. Alpha-internexin expression in gliomas: relationship with histological type and 1p, 19q, 10p and 10q status. J Clin Pathol 2011;64(9):793-801.

[61] Wan F, Herold-Mende C, Campos B, Centner FS, Dictus C, Becker N, Devens F, Mogler C, Felsberg J, Grabe N, Reifenberger G, Lichter P, Unterberg A, Bermejo JL, Ahmadi R. Association of stem cell-related markers and survival in astrocytic gliomas. Biomarkers 2011;16(2):136-43.

[62] Krupkova O, Jr., Loja T, Redova M, Neradil J, Zitterbart K, Sterba J, Veselska R. Analysis of nuclear nestin localization in cell lines derived from neurogenic tumors. Tumour Biol 2011;32(4):631-9.

[63] Nagaishi M, Yokoo H, Hirato J, Yoshimoto Y, Nakazato Y. Clinico-pathological feature of pilomyxoid astrocytomas: three case reports. Neuropathology 2011;31(2): 152-7.

[64] Yoshimoto K, Ma X, Guan Y, Mizoguchi M, Nakamizo A, Amano T, Hata N, Kuga D, Sasaki T. Expression of stem cell marker and receptor kinase genes in glioblastoma tissue quantified by real-time RT-PCR. Brain Tumor Pathol 2011;28(4):291-6.

[65] Idoate MA, Diez Valle R, Echeveste J, Tejada S. Pathological characterization of the glioblastoma border as shown during surgery using 5-aminolevulinic acid-induced fluorescence. Neuropathology 2011;31(6):575-82.

[66] Kim KJ, Lee KH, Kim HS, Moon KS, Jung TY, Jung S, Lee MC. The presence of stem cell marker-expressing cells is not prognostically significant in glioblastomas. Neuropathology 2011;31(5):494-502.

[67] Najbauer J, Huszthy PC, Barish ME, Garcia E, Metz MZ, Myers SM, Gutova M, Frank RT, Miletic H, Kendall SE, Glackin CA, Bjerkvig R, Aboody KS. Cellular host responses to gliomas. PLoS One 2012;7(4):e35150.

[68] He H, Li MW, Niu CS. The pathological characteristics of glioma stem cell niches. J Clin Neurosci 2012;19(1):121-7.

[69] Kong LY, Wu AS, Doucette T, Wei J, Priebe W, Fuller GN, Qiao W, Sawaya R, Rao G, Heimberger AB. Intratumoral mediated immunosuppression is prognostic in genetically engineered murine models of glioma and correlates to immunotherapeutic responses. Clin Cancer Res 2010;16(23):5722-33.

[70] Lu WJ, Lan F, He Q, Lee A, Tang CZ, Dong L, Lan B, Ma X, Wu JC, Shen L. Inducible expression of stem cell associated intermediate filament nestin reveals an important role in glioblastoma carcinogenesis. Int J Cancer 2011;128(2):343-51.

[71] Prestegarden L, Svendsen A, Wang J, Sleire L, Skaftnesmo KO, Bjerkvig R, Yan T, Askland L, Persson A, Sakariassen PO, Enger PO. Glioma cell populations grouped by different cell type markers drive brain tumor growth. Cancer Res 2010;70(11): 4274-9.

[72] Zhu G, Su W, Jin G, Xu F, Hao S, Guan F, Jia W, Liu F. Glioma stem cells targeted by oncolytic virus carrying endostatin-angiostatin fusion gene and the expression of its exogenous gene in vitro. Brain Res 2011;1390:59-69.

[73] Bulnes S, Garcia-Blanco A, Bengoetxea H, Ortuzar N, Argandona EG, Lafuente JV. Glial stem cells and their relationship with tumour angiogenesis process. Rev Neurol 2011;52(12):743-50.

[74] Xiao ZY, Tang H, Xu ZM, Yan ZJ, Li P, Cai YQ, Jiang XD, Xu RX. An experimental study of dendritic cells transfected with cancer stem-like cells RNA against 9L brain tumors. Cancer Biol Ther 2011;11(11):974-80.

[75] Tomuleasa C, Soritau O, Rus-Ciuca D, Ioani H, Susman S, Petrescu M, Timis T, Cernea D, Kacso G, Irimie A, Florian IS. Functional and molecular characterization of glioblastoma multiforme-derived cancer stem cells. J BUON 2010;15(3):583-91.

[76] Qin K, Jiang X, Zou Y, Wang J, Qin L, Zeng Y. Study on the proliferation and drug-resistance of human brain tumor stem-like cells. Cell Mol Neurobiol 2010;30(6):955-60.

[77] Michelakis ED, Sutendra G, Dromparis P, Webster L, Haromy A, Niven E, Maguire C, Gammer TL, Mackey JR, Fulton D, Abdulkarim B, McMurtry MS, Petruk KC. Metabolic modulation of glioblastoma with dichloroacetate. Sci Transl Med 2010;2(31):31ra4.

[78] Guo Y, Liu S, Wang P, Zhao S, Wang F, Bing L, Zhang Y, Ling EA, Gao J, Hao A. Expression profile of embryonic stem cell-associated genes Oct4, Sox2 and Nanog in human gliomas. Histopathology 2011;59(4):763-75.

[79] Wookey PJ, McLean CA, Hwang P, Furness SG, Nguyen S, Kourakis A, Hare DL, Rosenfeld JV. The expression of calcitonin receptor detected in malignant cells of the brain tumour glioblastoma multiforme and functional properties in the cell line A172. Histopathology 2012;60(6):895-910.

[80] Binello E, Qadeer ZA, Kothari HP, Emdad L, Germano IM. Stemness of the CT-2A Immunocompetent Mouse Brain Tumor Model: Characterization In Vitro. J Cancer 2012;3:166-74.

[81] Kim RK, Yoon CH, Hyun KH, Lee H, An S, Park MJ, Kim MJ, Lee SJ. Role of lymphocyte-specific protein tyrosine kinase (LCK) in the expansion of glioma-initiating cells by fractionated radiation. Biochem Biophys Res Commun 2010;402(4):631-6.

[82] Tamura K, Aoyagi M, Wakimoto H, Ando N, Nariai T, Yamamoto M, Ohno K. Accumulation of CD133-positive glioma cells after high-dose irradiation by Gamma Knife surgery plus external beam radiation. J Neurosurg 2010;113(2):310-8.

[83] Kolenda J, Jensen SS, Aaberg-Jessen C, Christensen K, Andersen C, Brunner N, Kristensen BW. Effects of hypoxia on expression of a panel of stem cell and chemoresistance markers in glioblastoma-derived spheroids. J Neurooncol 2011;103(1):43-58.

[84] Schiffer D, Annovazzi L, Caldera V, Mellai M. On the origin and growth of gliomas. Anticancer Res 2010;30(6):1977-98.

[85] Moon JH, Kwon S, Jun EK, Kim A, Whang KY, Kim H, Oh S, Yoon BS, You S. Nanog-induced dedifferentiation of p53-deficient mouse astrocytes into brain cancer stem-like cells. Biochem Biophys Res Commun 2011;412(1):175-81.

[86] Ying M, Wang S, Sang Y, Sun P, Lal B, Goodwin CR, Guerrero-Cazares H, Quinones-Hinojosa A, Laterra J, Xia S. Regulation of glioblastoma stem cells by retinoic acid: role for Notch pathway inhibition. Oncogene 2011;30(31):3454-67.

[87] Zarnescu O, Brehar FM, Bleotu C, Gorgan RM. Co-localization of PCNA, VCAM-1 and caspase-3 with nestin in xenografts derived from human anaplastic astrocytoma and glioblastoma multiforme tumor spheres. Micron 2011;42(8):793-800.

[88] He H, Niu CS, Li MW. Correlation between glioblastoma stem-like cells and tumor vascularization. Oncol Rep 2012;27(1):45-50.

[89] Dong J, Zhao Y, Huang Q, Fei X, Diao Y, Shen Y, Xiao H, Zhang T, Lan Q, Gu X. Glioma stem/progenitor cells contribute to neovascularization via transdifferentiation. Stem Cell Rev 2010;7(1):141-52.

[90] Natsume A, Kato T, Kinjo S, Enomoto A, Toda H, Shimato S, Ohka F, Motomura K, Kondo Y, Miyata T, Takahashi M, Wakabayashi T. Girdin maintains the stemness of glioblastoma stem cells. Oncogene 2012;31(22):2715-24.

[91] Maderna E, Salmaggi A, Calatozzolo C, Limido L, Pollo B. Nestin, PDGFRbeta, CXCL12 and VEGF in glioma patients: different profiles of (pro-angiogenic) molecule expression are related with tumor grade and may provide prognostic information. Cancer Biol Ther 2007;6(7):1018-24.

[92] Colman H, Zhang L, Sulman EP, McDonald JM, Shooshtari NL, Rivera A, Popoff S, Nutt CL, Louis DN, Cairncross JG, Gilbert MR, Phillips HS, Mehta MP, Chakravarti A, Pelloski CE, Bhat K, Feuerstein BG, Jenkins RB, Aldape K. A multigene predictor of outcome in glioblastoma. Neuro Oncol 2010;12(1):49-57.

[93] Lothian C, Lendahl U. An evolutionarily conserved region in the second intron of the human nestin gene directs gene expression to CNS progenitor cells and to early neural crest cells. Eur J Neurosci 1997;9(3):452-62.

[94] Birnbaum T, Hildebrandt J, Nuebling G, Sostak P, Straube A. Glioblastoma-dependent differentiation and angiogenic potential of human mesenchymal stem cells in vitro. J Neurooncol 2011;105(1):57-65.

[95] Matsuda Y, Fujii T, Suzuki T, Yamahatsu K, Kawahara K, Teduka K, Kawamoto Y, Yamamoto T, Ishiwata T, Naito Z. Comparison of Fixation Methods for Preservation of Morphology, RNAs, and Proteins From Paraffin-embedded Human Cancer Cell-implanted Mouse Models. J Histochem Cytochem 2010; 59 (1): 68-75.

[96] Yamahatsu K, Matsuda Y, Ishiwata T, Uchida E, Naito Z. Nestin as a novel therapeutic target for pancreatic cancer via tumor angiogenesis. Int J Oncol 2012; 40 (5): 1345-57.

[97] Mokry J, Nemecek S. Angiogenesis of extra- and intraembryonic blood vessels is associated with expression of nestin in endothelial cells. Folia Biol (Praha) 1998;44(5): 155-61.

[98] Mokry J, Nemecek S. Cerebral angiogenesis shows nestin expression in endothelial cells. Gen Physiol Biophys 1999;18 Suppl 1:25-9.

[99] Li MW, Niu CS. [Correlative study of distribution of brain tumor stem cell with micro-vascular system]. Zhonghua Yi Xue Za Zhi 2010;90(5):305-9.

[100] Sica G, Lama G, Anile C, Geloso MC, La Torre G, De Bonis P, Maira G, Lauriola L, Jhanwar-Uniyal M, Mangiola A. Assessment of angiogenesis by CD105 and nestin expression in peritumor tissue of glioblastoma. Int J Oncol 2011;38(1):41-9.

[101] Calabrese C, Poppleton H, Kocak M, Hogg TL, Fuller C, Hamner B, Oh EY, Gaber MW, Finklestein D, Allen M, Frank A, Bayazitov IT, Zakharenko SS, Gajjar A, Davidoff A, Gilbertson RJ. A perivascular niche for brain tumor stem cells. Cancer Cell 2007;11(1):69-82.

[102] Castino R, Pucer A, Veneroni R, Morani F, Peracchio C, Lah TT, Isidoro C. Resveratrol reduces the invasive growth and promotes the acquisition of a long-lasting differentiated phenotype in human glioblastoma cells. J Agric Food Chem 2011;59(8): 4264-72.

[103] Beck S, Jin X, Yin J, Kim SH, Lee NK, Oh SY, Kim MK, Kim EB, Son JS, Kim SC, Nam DH, Kang SK, Kim H, Choi YJ. Identification of a peptide that interacts with Nestin protein expressed in brain cancer stem cells. Biomaterials 2011;32(33):8518-28.

Permissions

The contributors of this book come from diverse backgrounds, making this book a truly international effort. This book will bring forth new frontiers with its revolutionizing research information and detailed analysis of the nascent developments around the world.

We would like to thank Dr. Terry Lichtor, for lending his expertise to make the book truly unique. He has played a crucial role in the development of this book. Without his invaluable contribution this book wouldn't have been possible. He has made vital efforts to compile up to date information on the varied aspects of this subject to make this book a valuable addition to the collection of many professionals and students.

This book was conceptualized with the vision of imparting up-to-date information and advanced data in this field. To ensure the same, a matchless editorial board was set up. Every individual on the board went through rigorous rounds of assessment to prove their worth. After which they invested a large part of their time researching and compiling the most relevant data for our readers. Conferences and sessions were held from time to time between the editorial board and the contributing authors to present the data in the most comprehensible form. The editorial team has worked tirelessly to provide valuable and valid information to help people across the globe.

Every chapter published in this book has been scrutinized by our experts. Their significance has been extensively debated. The topics covered herein carry significant findings which will fuel the growth of the discipline. They may even be implemented as practical applications or may be referred to as a beginning point for another development. Chapters in this book were first published by InTech; hereby published with permission under the Creative Commons Attribution License or equivalent.

The editorial board has been involved in producing this book since its inception. They have spent rigorous hours researching and exploring the diverse topics which have resulted in the successful publishing of this book. They have passed on their knowledge of decades through this book. To expedite this challenging task, the publisher supported the team at every step. A small team of assistant editors was also appointed to further simplify the editing procedure and attain best results for the readers.

Our editorial team has been hand-picked from every corner of the world. Their multi-ethnicity adds dynamic inputs to the discussions which result in innovative outcomes. These outcomes are then further discussed with the researchers and contributors who give their valuable feedback and opinion regarding the same. The feedback is then collaborated with the researches and they are edited in a comprehensive manner to aid the understanding of the subject.

Apart from the editorial board, the designing team has also invested a significant amount of their time in understanding the subject and creating the most relevant covers. They scrutinized every image to scout for the most suitable representation of the subject and create an appropriate cover for the book.

The publishing team has been involved in this book since its early stages. They were actively engaged in every process, be it collecting the data, connecting with the contributors or procuring relevant information. The team has been an ardent support to the editorial, designing and production team. Their endless efforts to recruit the best for this project, has resulted in the accomplishment of this book. They are a veteran in the field of academics and their pool of knowledge is as vast as their experience in printing. Their expertise and guidance has proved useful at every step. Their uncompromising quality standards have made this book an exceptional effort. Their encouragement from time to time has been an inspiration for everyone.

The publisher and the editorial board hope that this book will prove to be a valuable piece of knowledge for researchers, students, practitioners and scholars across the globe.

List of Contributors

Lee Roy Morgan
CEO DEKK-TEC, Inc. University of New Orleans New Orleans, LA, USA

P. O. Carminati, F. S. Donaires, P. R. D. V. Godoy and A. P. Montaldi
Department of Genetics, Faculty of Medicine of Ribeirão Preto, São Paulo University (USP), Ribeirão Preto, SP, Brazil

J. A. Meador and A.S. Balajee
Center for Radiological Research, Department of Radiation Oncology, College of Physicians and Surgeons, Columbia University, New York, NY, USA

G. A. Passos
Department of Genetics, Faculty of Medicine and Faculty of Dentistry, University of São Paulo, Ribeirão Preto, SP, Brazil.

E. T. Sakamoto-Hojo
Department of Genetics, Faculty of Medicine of Ribeirão Preto, São Paulo University (USP), Ribeirão Preto, SP, Brazil
Department of Biology, Faculty of Philosophy, Sciences and Letters of Ribeirão Preto, São Paulo University (USP), Ribeirão Preto, SP, Brazil

Chunzhi Zhang
Department of Radiation Oncology, Tianjin Huan Hu Hospital, Tianjin, China

Budong Chen and Jinhuan Wang
Department of Neurosurgery, Tianjin Huan Hu Hospital, Tianjin, China

Xiangying Xu, Baolin Han and Guangshun Wang
Department of Oncology, Tianjin Baodi Hospital, Tianjin, China

Sihan Wu, Wenbo Zhu and Guangmei Yan
Zhongshan School of Medicine, Sun Yat-sen University, People's Republic of China

Claudia C. Faria and James T. Rutka
Division of Neurosurgery and Labatt Brain Tumour Research Centre, the Hospital for Sick Children, University of Toronto, Canada

Christian A. Smith
Labatt Brain Tumour Research Centre, The Hospital for Sick Children, University of Toronto, Canada

Kristiina Nordfors
Department of Pediatrics, Tampere University Hospital, Tampere, Finland

Joonas Haapasalo
Unit of Neurosurgery, Tampere University Hospital, Tampere, Finland

Hannu Haapasalo
Department of Pathology, Fimlab Ltd and Tampere University Hospital, Tampere, Finland

Seppo Parkkila
Department of Anatomy, Tampere University, Fimlab Ltd and Tampere University Hospital, Tampere, Finland

P. R. D. V. Godoy, S. S. Mello and F. S. Donaires
Department of Genetics, Faculty of Medicine, University of São Paulo, Ribeirão Preto, SP, Brazil

E. A. Donadi
Department of Medic Clinic, Faculty of Medicine, University of São Paulo, Ribeirão Preto, SP, Brazil

G. A. S. Passos
Department of Genetics, Faculty of Medicine and Faculty of Dentistry, University of São Paulo, Ribeirão Preto, SP, Brazil

E. T. Sakamoto-Hojo
Department of Genetics, Faculty of Medicine, University of São Paulo, Ribeirão Preto, SP
Department of Biology, Faculty of Philosophy, Sciences and Letters-USP, University of São Paulo, Ribeirão Preto, SP, Brazil

Andrés Felipe Cardona
Clinical and Translational Oncology Group, Institute of Oncology, Fundación Santa Fe de Bogotá, Bogotá D.C., Colombia
Red LANO/ONCOL Group, Colombia

León Darío Ortíz
Red LANO/ONCOL Group, Colombia
Neuro-Oncology Group, Institute of Oncology, Clínicalas Américas, Medellín, Colombia

Yoko Matsuda, Hisashi Yoshimura, Taeko Suzuki and Toshiyuki Ishiwata
Departments of Pathology and Integrative Oncological Pathology, Nippon Medical School, Bunkyo-ku, Tokyo, Japan